Pelvic Inflammatory Disease and Chlamydia

A Guide to Causes, Treatment and Prevention

Patsy Westcott

Thorsons
An Imprint of HarperCollins*Publishers*

Thorsons
An Imprint of HarperCollins*Publishers*
77–85 Fulham Palace Road,
Hammersmith, London W6 8JB

Published by Thorsons 1992
1   3   5   7   9   10   8   6   4   2

A catalogue record for this book
is available from the British Library

ISBN 0 7225 2608 3

Typeset by Harper Phototypesetters Limited,
Northampton, England
Printed in Great Britain by
HarperCollinsManufacturing Glasgow

Pelvic Inflammatory Disease and Chlamydia

Contents

Chapter 1

'Am I Going Mad?'

The Victims

'I'd never even heard of Pelvic Inflammatory Disease until I had a terrible ectopic pregnancy three years ago and nearly died. No one told me what had caused it, or asked me about my previous medical history. It was only when I started to think back that I remembered having a severe vaginal infection over twelve years ago. I had to find out for myself what the possible causes could be. When I started digging around I discovered that I had had classical symptoms of Pelvic Inflammatory Disease.'

'I lived with two years of hideous pain. In that time I was forced to give up my job, my relationship cracked up, my children got tired of me always being ill, and I felt abandoned by the medical profession. I saw 23 doctors in all in a vain attempt to track down the cause of my condition. The last doctor I saw told me that my problem was all in my mind. I began to feel as though I was going mad.'

'I had my first attack after having a caesarean section and developing an abscess. For three years I was plagued by attacks of pain, vaginal discharge, and high temperature. Every time I went to my doctor he put me on antibiotics. I got very run-down because of all the medication, but the

7

doctor never told me I had PID. I'm a nurse and finally I asked him "Have I got PID?" He said "Yes, you probably have." End of story.'

'I developed problems after having my third child. At first it was just pain in my lower abdomen before my period. I put it down to pre-menstrual tension. The pain gradually got worse until I had to take a week off work every month because of it. My whole life seemed to revolve around my periods. Sex was unbearable and I was bleeding constantly between periods. My menstrual cycle went completely to pot. I tried everything: antibiotics, surgery, homoeopathy, herbs, but nothing touched it. All the doctor could suggest was a hysterectomy. Finally I collapsed and had to spend three weeks in bed. I was all right for a while and then I became ill again. Eventually, after being told that I would have to live with recurrent attacks unless I had a hysterectomy, I decided to go ahead. It seems to have solved the problem.'

'I'd never heard of Pelvic Inflammatory Disease until my partner and I decided to try for a baby and I discovered I was infertile. It was discovered during a laparoscopy that my tubes were completely blocked, and there was no chance of me conceiving naturally. I was told that I'd probably had an infection at some time in the past, but I don't remember it. I did used to suffer pain in the week or so before my period, and during the first few days of my period, but I put it down to PMT. We had five attempts at IVF (the test tube baby technique), without success. In the end I had to accept that I would never bear a child of my own.'

The Facts

Pelvic Inflammatory Disease – PID – is the name given to infection of the pelvic organs. Very often by the time a woman is aware that she has had it, it is too late. She tries for a baby and finds to her anguish that her tubes are irreparably blocked, or she becomes pregnant and the fetus implants in the tube, causing an agonizing and life-threatening miscarriage.

The fact is that every woman who is sexually active is at risk of Pelvic Inflammatory Disease. Yet, like those quoted above, few have even heard of the condition until they become victims. When they come to seek treatment they soon discover that many doctors are equally ignorant.

Another sad fact is that a lot of the suffering is unnecessary – if it is caught in the early stages, PID is almost always completely curable. To understand the scale of the problem and the impact it can have on a woman's life, consider these figures.

If you have a single attack of PID you have:

- Six to ten times the risk of another attack
- A one in six chance of infertility caused by blocked or damaged tubes – a risk that doubles with each subsequent attack
- Seven times the risk of an ectopic pregnancy (where the baby implants in the tube)
- A one in five chance of chronic pelvic pain
- A two in five chance of pain during lovemaking
- A four in five chance of period problems such as heavy periods, bleeding between periods and painful periods.

The Problem

The inflammation of PID is in fact the body's response to attack by invaders. Whenever the body is threatened by infection, blood rushes to the part under attack, carrying vital antibodies which cause swelling and heat in an attempt to quell the infection. It is the damage done by this natural protective mechanism which is responsible for the dire consequences of PID.

PID is a particularly insidious illness, because although you may have a dramatic attack with full-blown symptoms such as agonizing pain, swelling and high temperature, over half of all attacks are silent. They either produce no symptoms at all, or they are so slight that women don't seek help from their doctors. Just to complicate matters even further, the disease is incredibly difficult to diagnose. Even the most experienced doctors only get it right just over half of the time: the rest of the time the disease is mistaken for other problems such as irritable bowel syndrome or other gynaecological problems.

Perhaps the saddest fact of all is that teenagers and those at the beginning of their sex lives are most at risk – and yet they don't realize the consequences until much later, by which time the disease has taken its terrible toll. Many of these tragic consequences could be prevented if more people had access to simple information about what causes PID, how to avoid it, and how to recognize it so as to seek early treatment. Yet few of those who are most vulnerable know anything about the disease.

The outlook is equally bleak for sufferers. All too often they don't get the advice and help they need from the medical profession. They may endure long years of pain, uncomfortable sex and problems with their periods, without ever being told what is the matter. They may be prescribed endless courses of antibiotics that deplete their health, without having an adequate diagnosis. Their cries of distress go unheard or ignored, and sometimes they are told their symptoms are all in the mind. Even if they discover they are infertile, or suffer an ectopic pregnancy, no explanation may be offered as to why it happened.

A survey carried out by medical sociologist Patricia Weir in 1989 revealed the following.

● Medical treatment for PID is appalling. Most women receive no explanation for their condition and few are diagnosed straightaway, despite the fact that treatment is much more effective if the condition is treated early on.

- Diagnosis is poor and misdiagnosis is common. Few women are offered a laparoscopy – the only sure method of getting a definitive diagnosis.

- Fewer than 10 per cent of women are asked about their partner's medical history, despite the fact that in most cases the disease is sexually transmitted.

- Few women are warned that PID can be a long-term illness, so they don't know how they can deal with it.

The Size of the Problem

In industrialized countries it's estimated that ten to 13 out of every 1,000 women of childbearing age are victims of PID. The rate among 15 to 24-year-olds is even higher with around 20 sufferers per thousand. Put another way, 1 per cent of women aged 20 to 34 contract PID, and 2 per cent of teenagers. In the US 150 women a year die of the illness.

Alarming as these figures are, many experts believe that they are only the tip of the iceberg. For a start, they represent those women with PID who end up in hospital – a tiny minority. They don't include the many thousands who are treated by general practitioners, or in genito-urinary or gynaecological clinics, or those who never receive treatment at all because the disease is 'silent'. Even more worrying, the incidence of the disease is on the rise. US doctor Willard Cates, of the Centre for Disease Control, estimates that if present trends continue, by the year 2000 one in four women will be victims of PID.

The Mystery

PID, as we have seen, is on the increase – but why? Until recently the experts were puzzled. There was just one clue:

the inexorable rise of PID went hand in hand with the existence of modern methods of contraception such as the Pill, the IUD, and our more relaxed attitudes towards sex.

The obvious conclusion was that the disease was sexually transmitted in some way. It had long been recognized that the well-known STD (sexually transmitted disease) gonorrhoea was linked with PID, with one in five women who contracted gonorrhoea developing blocked tubes. But why, when gonorrhoea was on the decline, was PID still on the rise?

It was then that researchers highlighted a previously little regarded sexually transmitted disease called chlamydia.

Chlamydia is the most common STD in the world today. The organism that causes it is in fact a bacteria, and yet it behaves like a virus, hiding in the cells, where it may lie undetected for many years. In women, infection with chlamydia causes few or no symptoms. In men it is the cause of a mild urinary infection called non-gonococcal urethritis. Could this be the reason for the explosion in cases of PID? Sure enough, when researchers tested women with PID, their suspicions were proved correct. They discovered that between half and three-quarters had antibodies to chlamydia. Today chlamydia is recognized as the major cause of PID.

However, the story doesn't end there. It's now thought that chlamydia is not the sole culprit. There may be other factors involved, such as other organisms that live in the vagina. One of the reasons PID is so hard to treat is that doctors are still arguing about whether it is caused by a particular single organism or by many. Bacteria are crafty, and antibiotics that are effective against one type are often of no use in killing another. In the next few chapters we examine in more detail the symptoms of PID and look at the evidence incriminating chlamydia, how you can avoid it, and how you can get fast, effective treatment if you are at risk.

Chapter 2

Defining Pelvic Inflammatory Disease

It is confusing even to try to give a precise meaning for the term PID: there are many definitions and they are often used loosely. In practice PID is an umbrella term that embraces any inflammation in the upper genital tract and reproductive system. That is the cervix, or neck of the womb, the uterus, or womb, and the fallopian tubes, the two tubes which lead from the ovaries to the uterus.

Different terms may be used to describe your condition depending on the exact whereabouts of the infection. For example, there is cervicitis, when the infection has attacked the cervix; endometritis, when the inside of the uterus is affected; salpingitis, when the infection has penetrated as far as the fallopian tubes; oophoritis, when the ovaries are affected, and salpingo-oophoritis, when tubes and ovaries are infected.

There are varying grades of infection too, ranging from slight swelling and reddening through to a suppurating abscess. If the infection spreads, perhaps because of a burst abscess, it can lead to peritonitis, when the inside of the pelvic cavity becomes inflamed, or a condition called Fitzhugh-Curtis syndrome (perihepatitis) in which the tissues around the liver are affected.

Is It PID?

One of the problems of getting a diagnosis is the wide variety of symptoms PID can have. These can range from being so mild as to be virtually unnoticeable to being totally incapacitating. At one extreme you may notice a dull ache in your pelvis after making love that gets worse when you walk around. At the other you may collapse with a sudden attack of violent pain, and have to be rushed to hospital.

Pain in the lower abdomen is often the first clue. Sometimes this is followed by low backache, tiredness, raised temperature, vaginal discharge, bleeding, bloating or a feeling of fullness. Some women complain of nausea and vomiting.

However, very few sufferers suffer all the symptoms listed. In fact, according to the Canadian PID Society, only 16 per cent of women fit the classic textbook picture. PID is a complicated condition with many different causes. Many experts now believe that the symptoms vary depending on the precise cause.

As a rule of thumb, if you develop two or more of the symptoms listed, then see the doctor – especially if some or all of the symptoms come on at the same time.

Symptoms That Come On Suddenly

- High temperature (38°C/100°F or more) with a shivery feeling
- Pain during lovemaking (dyspareunia)
- Vaginal discharge which is unusual for you. It may be more copious than usual, or have an unusual smell or consistency
- Irregular bleeding or spotting in between periods or after sex
- Back pain

- Attacks of shaking.

Symptoms That Continue Over A Period Of Time

- Low backache or leg pain
- Weight loss or gain
- Nausea and dizziness
- Tiredness and depression
- Pain on passing water, wanting to pass urine more often, or feeling that you still want to pass more urine, even though you have emptied your bladder
- Painful periods
- General feeling of being under par
- Infertility or subfertility.

Plus

- Pelvic pain – occasional or constant pain in the lower abdomen to the centre and one or both sides. It can occur when you are making love, during a period or when you ovulate. The acid test is if a bimanual pelvic examination (internal) is painful. Some women also experience pain on passing water and opening the bowels.

Getting a Diagnosis

Because PID can present itself in so many different ways, getting an accurate diagnosis can be difficult. Margaret's story is typical.

'I had my first attack four and a half years ago when I was teaching in Germany. I started bleeding between periods, and went to the doctor who said I had cystitis and gave me antibiotics. However, the symptoms didn't clear up and a week later I went back in agony. My temperature was sky high and I was gushing blood. I was admitted to hospital with septicaemia and stayed there for a fortnight. The German doctors were unable to tell me what I had in English so it wasn't until I came back to England that I found out that I had PID.

'When I got home after that first attack I was still very ill, and in a huge amount of pain. I also had a lot of intestinal problems, such as diarrhoea, which I still have to this day. After two months' bed rest I still felt ghastly but I returned to work. I was experiencing extreme pain in my lower left side and bleeding between periods.

'Over the next 18 months I had three more attacks – I was in and out of hospital. If I went to the toilet I curled up because of the pain. The doctors didn't listen to me, but simply kept on prescribing more and more courses of antibiotics. By the time I'd finished with those I felt completely debilitated. I could hardly walk, and eventually I was forced to give up my teaching job. That's when the problems really started, because I had to get a medical diagnosis in order to claim early retirement benefit. I had endless swabs of tissue taken from my uterus, which was very painful, but no one could find any evidence of infection. I had blood tests, and numerous internals which I found very distressing.

'Even my family stopped taking me seriously after a while. My daughter, who is training to be a doctor, told me I had a seven-day illness that couldn't possibly be still affecting me after all that time. Finally I had a laparoscopy. The trouble was, although it showed scar tissue, it was only on the right side and I was experiencing pain on the left, so the doctor said she was unable to support my application for a pension. I'll never forget her words – she said "Well, there are adhesions there, but your pain is entirely on your left, and therefore your pain is imaginary. It's a bit like someone with an amputated limb." It was the end of the road. Ironically, six weeks ago I went for a check-up at the GU clinic and was told I had antibodies for chlamydia, and yet in all that time no one could find any evidence of infection.'

Misunderstood Or Mad?

Like Margaret, many victims of PID feel ignored or misunderstood by their doctors, their partners and by friends and relatives. You may be fobbed off, told that your symptoms are something you have to live with, or worse still, that they are all in your mind.

Jessica Pickard, who started the Pelvic Inflammatory Disease Support Group, says: 'My best achievement is probably convincing women with PID they are not alone. One woman told me that her greatest relief had come from knowing, now, that she wasn't being neurotic.'

An acute episode of PID can be dramatic and unmistakable. However, as we have seen, many cases of PID grumble on for years with only vague and unspecific symptoms that can be attributed to other conditions. For example, tiredness and a general feeling of being unwell are extremely common, especially among women. They are also symptoms of a host of other illnesses, including depression. Women are twice as likely to visit a doctor complaining of depression as men. However, once you are labelled as depressive it's hard to escape the label and get proper physical investigations carried out.

To make matters even more complicated, depression is likely to be a real factor. It's hardly surprising, given the debilitating symptoms of PID, if you do get depressed, especially if you can't get anybody to take your symptoms seriously!

Other symptoms such as the urinary symptoms can often be mistaken for cystitis, or other sexually transmitted diseases.

Types of PID

One of the problems with getting a diagnosis is that the experts disagree among themselves about the true nature of PID. Some experts define three different types of PID, according to how severe the infection is and how long it lasts. They are acute, recurrent and chronic (see box). However, such classifications are open to interpretation, and what one doctor may consider recurrent PID, another may define as the chronic variety. To make it even more complicated, some doctors don't use these terms at all. One of the biggest problems of all is that PID can often be subclinical: that is, it produces no symptoms whatsoever.

- **Acute PID.** This is when the infection comes on suddenly and violently. There is a high level of infection, and abscesses (pockets of pus) can form. If the abscess bursts, peritonitis (when the infection spreads to the lining of the abdominal cavity) can ensue – this is a potentially life-threatening condition.

- **Recurrent PID.** If the PID is left untreated, or is not treated properly, it may clear up of its own accord, but then come back again. Many women are plagued for years with recurrent attacks, especially when they are run down physically or emotionally. It's not known why this should happen, but it is thought that perhaps once the natural protective mechanisms have become broken down by a first attack of PID, the body is more susceptible to subsequent attacks. Recurrent PID can also result from failure of the original treatment to kill the infection fully. This can happen if the wrong antibiotics are used. Women can also become re-infected by their partners, which is

---

why it is important for both of you to be tested and treated.

- **Chronic PID.** When PID is untreated or inadequately treated it never clears up and the infection lingers on for long periods, causing discomfort but no acute pain. This is the most controversial diagnosis of all because some doctors say that, although a few women get accumulations of pus in the pelvis even after antibiotic treatment, chronic PID is actually very rare. They say that because antibiotics usually clear up the original infection, women who continue to suffer bouts of pain are in fact experiencing the effects of damage to the tissues done by the infection.

- **Subclinical PID.** When levels of infection are low there is less danger of an abscess forming. However, this type of PID is even more insidious and difficult to treat because it can grumble on for years without giving any problems, while all the time silently wreaking its damage. Subclinical PID can also flare up into an acute episode and lead to chronic pelvic pain, period problems, painful sex and all the other effects of acute PID.

What Causes PID?

The biggest cause of PID, as we saw in Chapter 1, is chlamydia, and the next chapter is devoted to the story of how doctors discovered chlamydia, and how to spot and treat it. However, we have not yet answered the question of how the infection which starts in the vagina reaches the pelvic organs.

Breaching the Cervical Barrier

The uterus or womb is completely sterile, sealed off from invading organisms by the cervix, or neck of the womb. In PID an infection such as chlamydia gets through the cervix and into the uterus, from where it travels to the other reproductive organs.

How does this happen? Under normal circumstances the opening of the cervix is tightly closed to prevent any foreign bodies from entering the sterile environment of the uterus. The cervix also produces mucus to stop infection getting through, and its cells secrete anti-infective agents which de-activate any micro-organisms before they can do any harm.

However, in certain circumstances the cervix becomes less able to carry out its protective function. Also, in some groups of women the body's defence system is not as efficient as it should be, making the cervix less able to protect them against the organisms that cause PID. Some of these circumstances are described below.

PID and Sex

The most common cause of pelvic inflammatory disease is, quite simply, making love. That's why it is absolutely vital for everyone who is sexually active to get checked out regularly for signs of infection.

Experts believe that between half and three-quarters of cases of PID are sexually transmitted. Many researchers believe the high rate of recurrent PID is a result of infection being passed backwards and forwards between partners: a theory that seems to be supported by some recent research from Sweden that shows that the more often you make love, the more at risk you are of contracting PID. In fact, those who make love an average of eight times a month or more have 10 to 20 per cent more episodes of PID than those who make love less often.

This seems to suggest that it's not simply 'promiscuity', as some researchers suggest, that leads to more PID, but that the spread of PID has something to do with the act of making love itself. One reason is that even though only certain micro-organisms are officially labelled sexually transmitted, in fact all sorts of other bacteria go backwards and forwards during sex.

Many of the organisms which cause infection aren't active enough to make their way up the vagina on their own, but they can do so on the back of sperm. Organisms such as the bacteria that cause gonorrhoea and chlamydia, another organism called *Ureaplasma urealyticum*, and several types of anaerobic bacteria – those that don't depend on oxygen in order to live – travel up the vagina in this way, and the contractions of the womb that happen during orgasm help draw them into the uterus.

There is another factor too. During lovemaking, pressure changes in the vagina cause the cervix to act like a mini-vacuum cleaner sucking up sperm into the body of the uterus. Anything that raises pressure in the vagina, for example water-skiing, can have a similar effect.

Number of Partners

Experts are still debating the role the number of sex partners you have has to play in your risk of PID. Several studies have shown that the more sex partners you have, the greater your risk of contracting PID. However, the most recent research suggests the case is not quite so clear-cut as that. Those who begin their sex lives early are likely to have had more sex partners than those who start later. And as I explain below, the earlier you start your sex life, the more likely you are to develop PID. The latest Swedish research shows that the link between the number of sex partners and PID disappears once the age factor is taken into account. The researchers say,

'[This] fact suggests that the time at which sexual life is initiated has more importance for PID than has the number of sexual partners in itself.'

Moral Panics

So the jury is still out on what effect the number of partners you have has to play in PID. Unfortunately, the very fact that PID is linked with sexual behaviour at all has led into a thicket of moral judgements which may affect the sort of reaction you get from medical staff and others. It's a sad fact that there is still a stigma attached to any disease which is perceived as being brought on by sexual activity. Some doctors – fortunately not those in most GU clinics – still take the attitude that 'you brought it on yourself'. This viewpoint may be particularly aimed at women because of the double standard which says that while it's OK for a man to have more than one sexual partner, women who do so are promiscuous or whores. Yet we have to have to accept that realistically speaking, few women these days go virgin to the altar. Moreover, the rising toll of divorce and separation means that many older women go on to have several more sexual relationships after a marriage ends. What is more, because the bacteria that cause the illness can often be symptomless, it's not just the number of partners a woman has which may facilitate the spread of PID, but the number a man has too.

As genito-urinary specialist Dr Patricia Munday pointed out in a talk to the British PID Society, 'People with STDs [sexually transmitted diseases] are entitled to just as much consideration, attention and kindness as are people with PID, AIDS, asthma or lung cancer. If you start saying ''we've got PID, we haven't got VD'', you are guilty of degrading STDs.'

Instead of stigmatizing those with PID – a factor which has helped keep it hidden from view, and hindered research into its causes – all of us need to be educated in safe sex practices to try and break the chain of infection.

Childbirth, Miscarriage, Caesarean Section and Abortion

During childbirth or miscarriage, for example, the cervix gradually dilates (is drawn up and stretches) to let the baby out. In an abortion instruments are used to surgically open the cervix, and the same happens during other surgical procedures such as a D and C (dilatation and curettage), or during the insertion of an IUD (intrauterine device). In a caesarean the surgeon cuts open the uterus in order to draw out the baby. All these procedures open the way for potential infection, which is why such care is taken to sterilize instruments and use aseptic techniques.

Once the cervical barrier has been breached in this way, infection is free to enter. Sometimes this infection is non-specific: that is, you haven't caught it from anybody else, but the bacteria have got in from outside. Sometimes, however, the procedure opens the way for an infection you already have outside the uterus, such as chlamydia, to enter. For example, the risk of developing PID after any abortion has been estimated as between 2 per cent and 5 per cent. But if you already have an infection at the time of the operation, you run ten times the risk of developing PID. Many experts believe that all centres offering abortion should screen women beforehand for chlamydia – one of the commonest underlying causes of PID. If this is not possible because of the time factor, preventive antibiotics should be given. Genito-urinary expert and gynaecologist Mr John Hare, of the Hinchinbrooke Hospital in Huntingdon, UK, says 'It's amazing that the vast majority of terminations are done without antibiotic cover'. He advises any woman about to undergo an abortion who has not been tested for chlamydia or offered antibiotics to ask if they will be given.

The Immune Connection

Childbirth, abortion and miscarriage are all potentially risky for another reason too. During pregnancy the immune system is depressed in order to prevent the mother's body from rejecting the baby, and this leaves the body more susceptible to infection. Some experts suggest that 15 per cent of tubal infections are due to post-delivery infection, especially with chlamydia. This is one of the main causes of secondary infertility – when a woman who has previously not had any problems conceiving becomes unable to do so.

Other factors may also weaken the immune system so it doesn't work as effectively. For example, the Pill dampens down the immune system, because it mimics pregnancy. This means that not only is the body less able to fight off infection, but any signs of infection are less likely to be obvious, because the symptoms of PID are actually caused, as we saw in Chapter 1, by the body's attempt to fight off the infection.

Teenage girls are at risk too, because the necks of their wombs contain fewer immune factors so they are less efficient at fighting off invaders. Mr John Hare explains: 'Once women become sexually experienced they build up anti-sperm antibodies, and general antibodies which neutralize the effects of infections. They also build them up with age. A teenage girl who has sex for the first time with a partner who has or who has had many other partners is far more prone to get a whole host of infections, because her resistance is virtually nil.'

Other factors which damage immunity come into it as well: stress, alcohol, smoking, drugs, eating the wrong foods and environmental pollution can all take their toll on the immune system, making the body less able to counter infection.

Many PID sufferers notice that they symptoms get worse

or they experience a flare-up if they are feeling run down or under par.

PID and Periods

Many women notice the symptoms of PID during a period or immediately afterwards, and sometimes the symptoms are confused with period pain. No one really knows why this should be the case, but it could be because the cervix opens slightly to allow the flow of menstrual blood through, and loses its normally protective plug of mucus. Another factor could be that the lining of the womb, which is shed during a period, normally offers some protection against invading bacteria. Thirdly, blood provides an ideal medium in which certain bacteria can flourish. Whatever the reasons, it's a good idea to use a condom or cap if you make love during a period.

Getting Through the Medical Maze

As we've seen, PID and chlamydia can be treated by many different doctors. One of the problems for women seeking treatment for PID is the lack of communication between doctors in different specialities. Unless you are attending for infertility treatment, you and your partner are likely to see different specialists. You may be referred to a gynaecologist, while your partner, if he has symptoms at all, is referred to a urologist.

Some urologists class bacteria that are capable of causing PID in women as 'normal', since they don't cause the man any problems. However, according to at least one leading US researcher, sperm samples should be completely free of bacteria. What's more, not all doctors perform bacteriological sperm tests – so a test that may show up the rogue bacteria is missed out altogether.

In an article in the US magazine *Healthsharing*, one sufferer describes how she did the round of 16 different doctors before she found a New York fertility specialist who thought to take swabs from her (symptomless) husband's urethra and cultured his sperm. She and her husband were treated with identical antibiotics effective against the range of bacteria found in both partners, and Debi was cured. However, she then had to undergo surgery to remove the scarring resulting from years of untreated infection. Her husband was lucky – antibiotics alone cured him.

The Age Factor

The earlier you start your sex life, the more likely you are to develop PID. Three-quarters of cases of PID occur in the under-25s – and teenagers are most at risk. Research shows that a sexually active 15-year-old has ten times more risk of developing the illness than her 25-year-old sister. Why? Well, for a start, at this age few women have entered a stable relationship, so you and any sexual partners you have are more likely to have other partners. Anyone who has several partners, or whose partner has several partners, is more at risk of contracting a sexually transmitted disease. At the same time, barrier methods of contraception, such as the cap and condom, which are known to protect against the organisms causing chlamydia, are less popular among this age group. What is more, the cells of the cervix are more delicate and prone to damage at this age, because they haven't yet built up the protective antibodies that more sexually experienced women produce. At this age too your hormonal system is undergoing a lot of upheaval. And though no one quite knows what role hormones have to play in PID, it is thought they have some influence in helping chlamydia, which as we've seen is one of the major causes of PID, to live longer. In fact, scientists wanting to grow chlamydia in laboratory animals actually feed them on the sex hormones oestrogen and progesterone in order to prolong the life of chlamydia. The hormone-influenced condition cervical erosion (known medically as ectopy), when cells from the inside of the cervix are formed on the outside, is more common at this age. And these cells are more susceptible to the bacteria which cause PID. For all these reasons, if you are in your teens and you think you might be at risk of PID, it's vital to go for regular checks to ensure you haven't contracted chlamydia.

Other Factors

There are various other lifestyle factors that may make you more vulnerable to PID. For example, those who smoke are twice as likely to develop PID as those who don't.

Douching, which is more widely practised in America than in the UK, is another risk factor, probably because of the pressure factor mentioned earlier and the risk of forcing organisms up through the cervix.

The Thrush Connection

Some researchers believe that thrush and other vaginal yeast infections can help the organisms causing PID to gain a foothold. It's thought that certain types of bacteria attach themselves to the yeast and travel up into the fallopian tubes. For this reason it pays to be on the lookout for any signs of vaginal infection and get them treated (see Preventing PID, page 100).

Am I At Risk?

Many experts have tried to quantify the various risk factors that make women more susceptible to PID. The trouble with this is that very often risk factors go together. For example, those who start their sex lives young (a known risk factor) are also more likely to have several sex partners (a more controversial risk factor), and not to use barrier methods of contraception (a known protective factor), so it is impossible to say whether a particular factor is a real risk or whether it appears to be because it is linked with another risk factor. The fact is that anyone who is sexually active is at risk of pelvic infection.

It's important to bear in mind too that when doctors talk about risk they are talking about groups of people based on statistics, and not about individuals. These are factors which have been found to be linked with a higher incidence of PID:

- Being in your teens and early twenties
- Beginning your sex life early
- Having an average of three or more sexual partners
- Type of contraception used. Using an IUD and using the Pill are linked with a higher incidence. Using barrier methods is linked with a lower incidence
- Having had an abortion or miscarriage
- Having had a previous pelvic infection or an infection following childbirth
- Having undergone gynaecological surgery or having had an injury to the vagina or cervix
- Having had other sexually transmitted diseases, or having a partner who has had other STDs
- Smoking
- Douching

Chapter 3

Chlamydia – The Silent Scourge

As we have seen, one of the major causes of PID is chlamydia. Until a few years ago chlamydia was not considered a particularly serious disease, partly because the organism itself is difficult to track down, and also because the disease it causes is so often symptomless – a fact which hinders diagnosis and helps spread infection – that doctors were unaware of the true extent of the problem and the amount of suffering it can cause.

Today chlamydia is recognized as the most common sexually transmitted disease in the West, with a whole cascade of potentially devastating consequences. Yet despite that, research into the disease is still insufficient and underfunded. One expert writing about the infection says, 'It is probable that we know less about chlamydia than about any other common, treatable pathogen.' *Intro.*

A Hidden Problem

One thing is certain: the chlamydia epidemic is of epic proportions. The disease is four times more common than it was 30 years ago. Accurate figures are hard to come by, because some cases are treated in genito-urinary clinics, some by family doctors or gynaecologists, and others never come to light at all, because the infection is silent. At least four out of ten cases of chlamydia detected in women attending STD clinics are symptomless. It's not surprising, then, that so many cases are either missed altogether or misdiagnosed.

In the United States it's estimated that three to four million people contract the infection each year. The latest British figures show that during the first nine months of 1988 90,000 cases of chlamydia were diagnosed in STD clinics – a third of them in women. However, chlamydia is crafty and can lie in hiding for many years, with the result that many cases are not diagnosed. Professor David Taylor-Robinson, head of research into sexually transmitted diseases at the Medical Research Council's Clinical Research Centre, Harrow, estimates that in women the true figures could be up to 30 per cent.

What Is Chlamydia?

Chlamydia is a type of bacteria. In parts of the Third World, untreated chlamydia is a leading cause of blindness, but in the West it is better known for its effects on the reproductive organs in both sexes, and the problems it can cause newborn babies.

In men, chlamydia can be responsible for the sexually transmitted illness non-gonococcal urethritis (NGU), and epididymitis (inflammation of the sperm duct), which is a major cause of male infertility. It can also lead to a type of arthritis.

In women, the infection, which begins in the cervix, can spread to the fallopian tubes. It is thought to account for between a quarter and a half of all cases of PID, especially endometritis (inflammation of the womb lining) and salpingitis (inflammation of the fallopian tubes). It also plays a part in cervicitis (inflammation of the cervix), and some of the tragic consequences of PID, ectopic pregnancy and infertility.

Alterations in hormone levels throughout the menstrual and reproductive cycle, or when you are on the Pill, can alter the surface of the cells and make them more favourable to chlamydia, making it easier for the organism to gain a foothold.

The effects of chlamydia also extend to the next generation. Women in the third stage of pregnancy are particularly vulnerable to chlamydia, because the immune system is dampened down during pregnancy, and they can pass it on to their babies. Babies born with chlamydia are at high risk of developing a virulent type of conjunctivitis, upper respiratory infections, and pneumonia. Tragically, they also have an increased risk of perinatal mortality (infant death).

Facts and Figures

To give some idea of the scale of the problem, take the following figures: in one London genito-urinary clinic 71 per cent of women with pelvic inflammatory disease, 68 per cent of men with NGU, 50 per cent of newborn babies with conjunctivitis, 47 per cent of women with cervicitis and vaginal discharge, and 46 per cent of contacts of men with NGU were found to have chlamydial infection.

The Chlamydia Organism

Although chlamydia is officially a bacteria – it has cell walls, divides by binary fission, and is sensitive to antibiotics – it behaves more like a virus. It is tiny and is able to hide among its host cells, so that it can lie undetected for months or years. Like a virus, too, it relies on its host cells for energy and can only reproduce inside living cells.

There are two different species of chlamydia. *Chlamydia*

psittaci causes psittacosis, which is a disease transmitted to humans from infected birds and sheep. But the one that is responsible for PID is called *Chlamydia trachomotis*.

The organism often lies dormant until it is triggered off by another genital infection or by a change of partner. More relaxed attitudes to sex, and the fact that the illness is frequently without symptoms, mean it is on the increase. The organism is difficult and expensive to culture, so routine screening is not performed. What's more, few people are aware of the disease and its potentially serious consequences.

A Medical Detective Story

In fact, although chlamydia has only recently hit the headlines, it has been known about since the beginning of this century.

The story of chlamydia and medicine begins in 1909, when it was first recognized as a source of eye infections in newborn babies and adults. By 1911 it was known that the same organism could infect the urethra in men, and the cervix in women. However, it wasn't until the late 50s and early 60s, when scientists developed more sophisticated techniques for isolating chlamydia, that the true extent of the damage it could wreak began to be revealed.

The Male Connection

The first big breakthrough came when it was discovered that chlamydia was the culprit in half of all cases of a sexually transmitted disease affecting men known as non-gonococcal urethritis (NGU). The illness used to be known as non-specific urethritis (NSU), because the cause was not known. Although NGU can have other causes, it is now known that chlamydia is responsible for up to half of all cases.

The latest studies show that chlamydia can be isolated from

the cervix of six to seven out of ten of the sexual partners of men with chlamydial NGU.

NGU can cause discharge from the penis and stinging or burning on passing urine. However, often men miss out on treatment because they have no symptoms. In this way they pass the disease on their partners, who may themselves in turn have no symptoms. In this way a chain of infection is created, putting both carriers and those they infect at risk of the serious consequences. Worse still, many doctors still consider NGU a trivial disease. Only a few GU clinics attempt to trace partners of patients being treated for the disease, and family doctors are even less likely to have the time or facilities to allow them to follow up contacts.

Cervicitis and Cervical Ectopy

Cervicitis simply means inflammation of the cervix, or neck of the womb. Normally the tough outer cells of the cervix protect it against infection. However, the cervix can become vulnerable to infection through trauma caused by an IUD or by vigorous love-making, or if you have an erosion, known medically as an ectopy. An erosion happens when some of the delicate cells from inside the womb grow on the outside, forming a soft reddened area. An erosion is usually quite painless, and doesn't create any trouble unless it becomes infected. In fact, if you have one you probably won't know until a doctor points it out during an internal examination.

Erosions can develop as a result of hormonal changes during pregnancy, when taking the Pill or at other times of hormonal upheaval. Symptoms of cervicitis, or when an erosion has become infected, include bleeding after sex, and a mucus discharge which may be offensive.

Doctors are still debating whether chlamydia is a cause of cervicitis, or whether the cells of the cervix become more susceptible to chlamydia when an erosion is present.

However, scientists have discovered more chlamydia in women with cervicitis than in those whose cervixes were normal. In one study of women attending an STD clinic most of those who were chlamydia-positive had some abnormality of the cervix, such as cervicitis or a cervical erosion.

Chlamydia and Cervical Smears

The smear test picks up abnormalities in the cells of the cervix, some of which can, if left untreated, lead on to cervical cancer. Women who began their sex lives early and those who have had several sex partners, or whose partners have had several sex partners, are more at risk of developing such abnormalities.

Antibodies to chlamydia have been found in four out of ten women with abnormal cervical smears, compared to only two out of ten of those with no changes in cell tissue.

However, the links between an abnormal smear and chlamydia are far from being clear-cut. A recent study carried out in Glasgow comparing women with normal and abnormal smears found a high incidence of chlamydia in both groups. The same study also discovered a high rate of previous infection in both groups of women.

Chlamydia and Other Sexually Transmitted Diseases

Sexually transmitted diseases tend to go together. Chlamydia, for example, has a particular affinity for gonorrhoea. Although gonorrhoea is far less common these days than it used to be, about 20 per cent of men and a third of women with gonorrhoea are also infected with chlamydia. Like all STDs, chlamydia is also more common in those developing HIV. If you suspect you have put yourself at risk of contracting HIV it is worth getting a chlamydia test, even if you decide not to be HIV tested. If you do have HIV you need to build up your strength and be free of infections to stay as healthy as possible for as long as possible.

If you have chlamydia or think you could have another sexually transmitted disease, it's worth getting a comprehensive screening at your local GU clinic to make sure that everything has been cleared up.

Chlamydia and Gynaecological Operations

Chlamydia can be carried into the womb on surgical instruments used to open the cervix during an abortion, or any surgical procedure in which the cervix is opened. The environment of the uterus provides the perfect medium for the bacteria to grow, especially if the abortion is incomplete and any tissues are left behind.

Chlamydia, PID and Infertility

The link between chlamydia and PID was first observed in the 1930s, when it was noticed that mothers of babies with eye infections were more likely to have PID. By 1975 a scientist had revealed anti-chlamydia antibodies in women with PID.

One famous Swedish study showed that of 20 women with PID, the fallopian tubes of six of them were infected by chlamydia, and 19 of 53 had cervical infections. Today, definite links are recognized between previous infection with chlamydia and abnormalities of the fallopian tubes in women attending infertility clinics. Yet still far too few clinics follow up contacts of patients with chlamydia.

Dr Patricia Munday, a consultant genito-urinary physician who has a special interest in chlamydia, believes that if clinics traced the contacts of patients with NGU it would have a major impact on tubal infertility. 'Doctors think if it is not gonorrhoea, it is not serious,' she says.

Am I At Risk?

Anyone who is sexually active is at risk of contracting chlamydia. The illness certainly isn't choosy about who it picks on. However, certain groups do have a higher incidence of the disease. They include young women under 24, young men, and those who have several sex partners. The rate of infection for sexually active women under 20 is two to three times higher than the rate for those aged 20 to 29.

Because it can lie dormant for many years without causing any problems, many cases occur even in stable relationships, where both partners are faithful. Unfortunately, the fact that chlamydia is associated with sexual promiscuity in some minds is one reason why it has remained in the shadows for so long. Doctors often don't test for chlamydia on the assumption that 'Nice girls don't get sexually transmitted diseases'. For this reason many experts argue that everyone who is sexually active should go for regular check-ups.

Who Gets Chlamydia?

Although chlamydia can strike anyone, certain groups are more at risk – possibly because their lives means they are more likely to be exposed to infection. They include:

● Those under 24
● Single men and women of any age
● Those using the Pill or no contraception
● Those in lower social groups
● Those who have had a new partner within the last two months
● Those living in towns and cities.

The incubation period for chlamydia is five to ten days or longer. Signs include:

- Discharge from the vagina, or urethra – the tube that leads from the bladder – in men
- Burning on passing water
- Pain in the testicles in men
- Bleeding or pain on making love
- Irregular periods
- Pain or discharge in the rectum (back passage).

It is important to realize that you may have some or all of these symptoms or none at all. One study found that a third of women who were chlamydia positive had no symptoms.

Diagnosis

Diagnosis involves discovering antibodies to chlamydia, using a variety of methods. A sample of mucus is taken from the cervix (just like having a cervical smear) or from the urethra in men. Unfortunately, despite the fact that chlamydia is so common, facilities for testing are woefully inadequate. In 1987, when the British Royal College of Physicians' committee on genito-urinary medicine surveyed the availability of chlamydia diagnosis in the UK and Ireland, they found that eight consultants in GU medicine had no access to chlamydia diagnostic facilities. Others were limited to screening women, and others only to screening those at high risk. Another problem until recently has been the insensitivity of most diagnostic techniques.

Cell culture, where a sample of mucus or blood is cultured in the laboratory, is considered to be the most reliable test. However, the process is long-winded – it takes at least 48 hours for the bacteria to multiply enough to be seen under a microscope – and costly. Even then the test is not always accurate. Sometimes the cervix produces neutralizing antibodies so that chlamydia is missed. And much can depend too on the skill of the doctor taking the sample, and the scientists culturing it.

Another method, known as direct immunofluorescence testing, detects the presence of chlamydia by means of an antibody reaction. The sample is mixed with a fluorescent dye which sticks to the chlamydia particles, allowing them to show up under a special microscope. The technique is fast, but the production and preparation of samples is time-consuming, and the accuracy of tests can vary depending of the skill of the technician performing the test.

Yet another test called ELISA, short for enzyme-linked immunosorbent assay, tests for a reaction between enzymes and antibodies specific to chlamydia which produce a colour signal. The test is simple and cheap. These tests can be highly automated and quick, and because they don't involve scientists using their own judgement to interpret the result, they are less open to the charge of human error, although inaccuracies can still creep in.

In Bristol, researchers are working on a simple urine enzyme test which would cut out the need to take urethral samples from men, which can sometimes be uncomfortable or painful. So far the test has proved quick and accurate. However, there is no equivalent test for women, and many GPs don't have the facilities for testing, and have to send samples to already overloaded laboratories. There is also the danger that chlamydia doesn't survive the journey and the test comes back negative, even though you have chlamydia.

Should I Be Screened?

Given the difficulties and limitations of the various diagnostic tests, it's clearly not practical for everyone to be tested for chlamydia. What's more, in Britain NHS laboratories couldn't cope with the load on their services if mass screening were introduced. However, many experts believe a limited screening service should be available. In Sweden, for example, all women about to have an abortion, those seeking contraceptive advice, and those with a vaginal discharge are routinely screened. As a result, the number of teenage girls with chlamydia has dropped by over half in the last five years.

Professor David Taylor Robinson believes all women attending STD clinics, those about to undergo an abortion, and pregnant women who are nearing term should be screened.

In the meantime, until the powers that be can be persuaded to introduce screening, it's up to women themselves to take charge of their own health, and make sure they are well-informed. Anyone who is sexually active would be wise to attend for regular check-ups, especially if they take on a new partner.

Your local genito-urinary clinic is more likely than your GP to have the equipment and facilities for proper diagnosis and contact tracing. However, with increased knowledge about chlamydia, government encouragement for GPs to carry out more tests themselves, and the existence of cheaper simpler tests, some GPs do now have facilities for testing.

Many GU clinics have walk-in sessions, where you can be seen straightaway. At others you need to make an appointment. You'll find the telephone number of your nearest clinic in the Yellow Pages under the name of your local hospital – after that it may list special clinic, GU clinic or even, in some areas still, VD clinic. Alternatively, ring the hospital switchboard and ask for the GU or special clinic. You will have to answer some questions about your sex life. Don't be daunted by this, or let it put you off seeking treatment. There is nothing to be embarrassed or ashamed of: the staff in GU clinics are experienced both in asking questions and performing examinations, and think no more of it than if they were examining you for a sore throat or asking you who you caught athlete's foot from.

Treatment

Once diagnosis has been carried out, treatment is simple and effective. A seven-day course of an antibiotic such as tetracycline is the most usual treatment. Tetracycline shouldn't be taken if you are pregnant, as it can affect the developing baby, so it's important to use a reliable contraceptive while you are taking it. The drug can also make you sensitive to the sun. It's vital to take the treatment exactly as prescribed on an empty stomach.

Erithromycin is an alternative for those who are pregnant, are allergic to tetracycline or can't avoid sun exposure, for example because they have an outdoor job.

In men a new drug called azithromycin which is taken in a single dose is being tested with some promising results. Many of these drugs are extremely strong and, not surprisingly, they may have side-effects including stomach upsets and allergy. Ask the doctor beforehand what you might expect in the way of reactions, and report back if they do have an adverse effect. Some should not be taken by people suffering from liver or kidney disease. And make sure the doctor knows if you are pregnant or breastfeeding a baby. For a final double check read the packet insert when you pick up your prescription.

Some doctors believe that, since chlamydia so often travels side by side with gonorrhoea, all those who are positive for gonorrhoea should also be treated for chlamydia, whether the infection is confirmed by a lab test or not. Penicillin, the treatment for gonorrhoea, doesn't cure chlamydia.

Action Plan

● Chlamydia, like all sexually transmitted diseases, is less common if you use a barrier method of contraception such as condoms or caps and spermicide. If you have more than one sex partner, or believe your partner has more than one sex partner, it's safer healthwise to use a condom and a spermicide.

● Go for regular testing every year, or whenever you change your partner. Find out beforehand whether the clinic you are planning to attend screens for chlamydia – not all of them do – and if possible go somewhere else if they don't have facilities for testing.

● If your partner has symptoms such as discharge from the penis or urinary symptoms, make sure you are tested and treated too – even if you don't have any symptoms.

● If you are found to be chlamydia positive, make sure your partner is treated – even if he has no symptoms – or you could be re-infected.

● If you aren't in a one-to-one relationship and the clinic you attend does not do contact tracing, get in touch with any recent partners yourself. Only in this way can the chain of infection be broken.

Chapter 4

Other Causes

The discovery that chlamydia is the prime cause of PID has led to less emphasis being placed on other causes of the condition. But it's still important to be aware of these, since they will affect treatment, and will also affect the symptoms of PID.

The Contraceptive Conundrum

The precise relationship between PID, chlamydia and contraceptives is a complicated one, and experts are still arguing about the part contraceptives have to play in the development of PID. One thing is certain: barrier methods of contraception such as the condom (sheath) and the diaphragm have a protective effect. The case for the Pill and the IUD is more murky.

The Pill Story

For a long time experts have been claiming that the Pill protects against PID. Three possible mechanisms have been suggested. Firstly, the Pill thickens the cervical mucus, creating a physical barrier to certain micro-organisms, such as those causing gonorrhoea, which don't live inside living cells. Secondly, it seems to decrease the muscular activity of the womb, so preventing the propulsion of microbes into the cervix. Thirdly, gonorrhoea organisms multiply in blood, so because the Pill cuts the amount of blood loss during a period, it is more difficult for the organism to flourish.

Unfortunately the case, as always with PID, isn't that clear-cut. There are other factors to consider. For a start, those experts who claim a protective effect from the Pill are basing their claim on the number of cases of PID admitted to hospital, and as we have seen, most cases of PID are not treated in hospital. Secondly, as we have also seen, the Pill suppresses the immune system with the result that PID is more likely to be subclinical and to produce no symptoms. Just because the PID doesn't produce symptoms doesn't mean, of course, that it can't lead to infertility, though the inflammatory changes in women on the Pill are usually not so marked, and Pill-users have been found to be less likely to develop severe salpingitis (inflammation of the fallopian tubes). Thirdly, as we have seen chlamydia, unlike gonorrhoea, lives inside cells, so the thick mucus will have no protective effect. What is more, women on the Pill are more likely to have a cervical erosion (ectopy) because of hormones involved in the Pill, and as we have also seen, the cells from the inside of the uterus are more vulnerable to chlamydia. Some studies show that Pill-users are slightly more likely to develop cervicitis (infection of the cervix).

Another confusing factor is that most studies of the Pill as a protective factor for PID were looking at old-fashioned high-dose oestrogen Pills which are now no longer used.

Results are conflicting and confusing. Some studies done in STD clinics appearing to show that the Pill boosts the risk of contracting chlamydial PID, but lowers the risk of PID caused by gonorrhoea. Other research shows that the Pill protects against the development of PID in those already infected with chlamydia, but not with gonorrhoea. Interpretation of the results is made even more difficult by the fact that there may be other confounding factors linked with Pill use which are also risk factors for PID, such as number of partners, frequency of love-making, smoking, and so on.

It's all very confusing, so what are we to make of it all? The very latest research seems to show that low dose forms of the Pill may protect against the most severe cases of PID that require hospital treatment. On the latest evidence progestogen-only types of Pill (the mini-Pill) seem to offer no particular protection against PID. Clearly, more research is needed into the effect of different types of Pill on PID, and also the effect of the Pill on infertility caused by blocked or damaged tubes.

IUD Dilemmas

So the jury is still out on the Pill, but what about the IUD? Experts have long pointed to the IUD as a risk factor for the development of PID. At a major conference on PID in 1980, one paper showed that IUD users were 10 times more likely to get PID than those using other methods of contraception. Since then, 25 separate studies have showed a link between IUDs and PID or tubal infertility. It was suggested that micro-organisms travel into the womb up the strings which hang out of the device. In particular, the Dalkon Shield IUD was found to boost the risk of PID five times more than other IUDs. The Dalkon Shield is now no longer available following massive court cases in America.

However, according to the latest studies, the evidence incriminating the IUD in PID is not as strong as it once seemed. For a start, the IUDs used today are medicated (copper containing), whereas the ones used in earlier studies showing an increased risk of PID were unmedicated. The

Oxford Family Planning Study Report of 1990 – a large long-term study into different types of contraception – showed that medicated devices carry only half the risk of non-medicated devices. However, why increase the risk at all? The study also showed that fertility rates after the removal of IUDs are remarkably high, a finding you wouldn't expect if IUDs caused PID. Another study, this time carried out in America, showed that once you take into account lifestyle, and the presence of antibodies to chlamydia, the link between IUDs and PID is lost. Women with only one sex partner using IUDs had no increased risk of tubal infertility.

Again, more research is desperately needed, but what the evidence seems to boil down to is that those in faithful one-to-one relationships who use an IUD are no more likely than anyone else to develop PID. Where the risk comes in is where an IUD is inserted when the woman is already infected with chlamydia, or where she is at risk of contracting chlamydia, because she or her partner has other partners. The IUD works by irritating the lining of the uterus, so making the tissue more prone to infection. The risk of developing PID seems to be higher in the first month or so after insertion, suggesting that infection is carried up into the uterus and tubes by the procedure. The lesson here is when choosing which contraception to use, look at yourself and your lifestyle. A recent American review advises, 'White women aged 25 years or older, who have only one sex partner and have intercourse five or fewer times a week, can be expected to have little risk of PID.' If you are not in a stable one-to-one relationship then the IUD is not for you. Even if there is any hint that you could be infected with chlamydia, tests should be taken, and the IUD inserted at a later date after results have proved negative or you have been treated.

Other Sexually Transmitted Diseases Besides Chlamydia

Gonorrhoea

Until the 1970s, gonorrhoea was considered to be the main cause of PID. Today, although chlamydia is thought to be the most common cause of PID, gonorrhoea is still important, especially as it often goes hand in hand with chlamydia, and also because PID caused by gonorrhoea is more likely to result in infertility.

It's estimated that between 10 and 19 per cent of women who have had gonorrhoea develop PID, and of these women between 15 and 40 per cent become sterile after just one attack.

What Is It?

Gonorrhoea is one of the oldest sexually transmitted diseases, affecting about 25,000 women a year in the UK. It is caused by the gonococcus bacteria. It can infect the urethra (the tube that leads from the bladder), the Bartholin's glands, which lie at the entrance to the vagina, the cervix, and the throat (if you have had oral sex with a sufferer). It can also infect the rectum (back passage) even if you haven't indulged in anal sex. The illness can be spread during ordinary intercourse, anal sex or oral sex. It can also be passed on through non-sexual contact with a gonorrhoea sufferer.

For example, mothers can pass it on to their babies during birth, or children can contract the illness by using a towel or flannel that has recently been used by a sufferer. (However, most cases in children are through sexual abuse.) If it spreads to the eyes it can cause a serious type of conjunctivitis, which can, if left untreated, lead to blindness.

What To Look Out For

One of the problems with gonorrhoea, as with chlamydia, is that it is often symptomless in men and in women, until it spreads and causes PID. Studies show that between four and six women out of ten don't notice symptoms of gonorrhoea, or confuse them with another illness.

Where symptoms do appear, they develop between two days and three weeks after making love with an infected person. You may notice an increase in vaginal discharge which may in addition be offensive and yellow. Pain on passing water, and wanting to pass urine frequently (urethritis) are other common symptoms, which can be mistaken for cystitis. The Bartholin's glands, which lie on either side of the vagina and provide lubrication when you are sexually aroused, can become swollen.

If you have had oral sex with a sufferer you may have a sore throat and swollen glands; these, of course, can easily be confused with a throat infection. If the rectum becomes infected, either by the vaginal discharge or through anal intercourse, you may notice itchiness in the back passage, discharge and pain when you open your bowels.

A small minority of sufferers – about 3 per cent – develop what is known as disseminated gonococcal infection, when the bacteria get into the circulation and attack the heart valves, which causes a form of meningitis. Symptoms include a rash, shiveriness, raised temperature, joint pain and pain in the tendons of the hand.

If the illness is left untreated and spreads to cause PID, you may have pain on one or both sides of the abdomen, vomiting, a raised temperature, bleeding from the vagina, spotting between periods or irregular periods, and/or a swollen abdomen.

Your Partner

In men the infection can attack the urethra, and can spread to the testicles where it causes swelling and pain. Left untreated, it can cause narrowing of the urethra, making it difficult and painful to pass water. Tragically, gonorrhoea frequently has no symptoms in women until it has done irreversible damage to the fallopian tubes. For this reason, your only clue may be if your partner has symptoms. In men, symptoms include a discharge from the penis and pain on passing water. If you know that your partner has a penile discharge, insist that he is tested for gonorrhoea so you can both be treated as soon as possible.

Diagnosis

Gonorrhoea is best treated in a GU clinic where facilities for rapid and accurate diagnosis are available. However, as with chlamydia, testing can take time, and results are not always accurate. Two main types of test may be used; both involve taking a sample of the cervical discharge (or urethral in men). Samples may also be taken from the anus (don't be embarrassed about having this done – as far as the doctor is concerned it is a routine measure that he or she thinks no more of than, say, peering into your ears if you had an ear infection), or from the throat. Women who have had a hysterectomy should have a urethral sample taken – this takes a couple of seconds. It doesn't hurt, but it may be momentarily mildly uncomfortable.

Cell culture, the most reliable test, involves incubating the sample for up to two days. The test is usually accurate when performed in a GU clinic where all facilities are on site. If your own doctor carries out the test it is much less accurate, as specimens can be damaged in transit.

The other test, known as the gram stain test, can be done on the spot. It is highly accurate for men with symptoms, but less good at picking up the bacteria in women and men without symptoms. A smear of discharge is stained with a special dye that shows up the gonorrhoea bacteria under a microscope.

It's worth finding out which test has been done, as accuracy varies greatly. The gram stain test is only 50 per cent accurate for women and men without symptoms, whereas the cell culture test is 90 per cent accurate, when the cells are taken from the cervix and anus. If your partner's test shows up positive, it is worth being treated, even if your test is negative. And if the initial test is negative, but you know you have definitely been exposed to the disease, it's also worth being treated.

Treatment

Once the result of your test is known, treatment with antibiotics can start. However, if you have had the cell culture test, some doctors like to start treatment straight away without waiting for the results to come back. There are pros and cons to this. On the one hand, the sooner the disease is treated the better, and the less likelihood there is of it spreading and causing PID. On the other hand, it's not a good idea to take unnecessary antibiotics, for all sorts of reasons. Another problem is that chlamydia can sometimes be confused with gonorrhoea, but chlamydia is treated with the antibiotic tetracycline, whereas gonorrhoea is treated with penicillin. If you are being treated for gonorrhoea, you should always ask to be tested and treated for chlamydia too, since treating gonorrhoea alone may mask chlamydia, with the subsequent risk of PID developing.

Treatment usually involves either injections of high doses of penicillin, or taking high-dose tablets of ampicillin, or a combination of the two. While you are being treated you shouldn't drink alcohol, as it can cause a nasty reaction. You may also be given another drug which helps the antibiotics to remain longer in your bloodstream. If you are allergic to penicillin, alternative medication can be given. One of the biggest problems with gonorrhoea is that penicillin-resistant strains have developed. If tests show that the type of gonorrhoea you have is of this variety another drug, such as spectinomycin, will be prescribed.

Follow-on Tests

To ensure that you are completely cured, and that no pockets of infection that could cause further problems remain, you will need to have further culture tests done. If they are still positive you will be treated with a different antibiotic, and a test should be done to see if the variety of the disease you have is penicillin-resistant. It's also vital that your partner should be tested and treated too, so that you don't become reinfected.

Other Bacteria

The list of bacteria thought to be involved in causing PID is steadily growing, and more are still being discovered. Not all of these bacteria are sexually transmitted in the sense in which we normally understand the term, although some of them may be transported to the reproductive organs by sperm. Others travel with yeast infections such as thrush, or on their own by a process known as passive transport.

These organisms are a mixture of anaerobic bacteria (so called because they can't live without oxygen) and aerobic bacteria (which need oxygen in order to survive). Some of these bacteria, such as *E coli*, normally live in the back passage and the gut without causing any problems. If they spread to the vagina or the bladder during sex, or through inadequate hygiene, they can be responsible for cystitis.

According to Swedish research, about 5 per cent of cases

of PID are caused by these 'normal' flora. This type of PID often comes on suddenly and with severe symptoms, such as a raised temperature and abscesses. Women suffering with this type of PID also tend to be older and have had chronic PID symptoms, or have had two or more attacks of the illness. It's thought that in these cases an initial attack of PID has damaged the protective mechanisms of the fallopian tubes, making them more vulnerable to subsequent infection.

PID and Other Vaginal Infections

This is an umbrella term for a group of vaginal infections that used to be known as non-specific vaginitis. Today more and more of the organisms that cause them are being identified as causes of PID, either alone or in combination with chlamydia. Many of them are anaerobic.

Mycoplasmas

In particular, a type of anaerobic bacteria known as *Mycoplasma hominis* is believed to be the culprit in between one and two in ten cases of PID. Like chlamydia, it is a cross between a virus and a bacteria. The organisms live in the vagina or cervix and can be found in the urethras of men with NGU. Symptoms are a watery, fishy-smelling discharge which often gets worse after making love. If untreated, as well as causing PID, the organism can also be responsible for premature birth and postnatal complications. However, although mycoplasmas are potentially so serious, not all clinics have facilities for testing for them.

Treatment is with an antibiotic, such as metronidazole (Flagyl) or amoxyllin, which should be taken by both partners.

Another type of mycoplasma, confusingly known as *Ureaplasma urealyticum*, may also be involved in PID – though doctors are still arguing as to whether it is actually a cause, or whether it simply appears to be involved because it often travels with chlamydia. The organism can cause a urinary infection, with symptoms similar to chlamydia, and causes up to a quarter of cases of NGU in men. It is frequently found in the genital tracts of people who are apparently healthy, without giving rise to any symptoms. Treatment is with tetracycline, but some strains are resistant to the antibiotics, so a follow-up check to make sure treatment has worked is vital.

A micro-organism called *Actinomyces*, a cross between a bacteria and a fungus, has come under increasing suspicion of causing PID, especially in women who have an IUD. The germ has to enter the body through a mucous membrane, such as those found in the mouth or the genital tract. The subsequent infection, known as actinomycosis, causes pussy abscesses.

How to Avoid Vaginal Infections

Because of the potentially serious consequences of any vaginal infections, you should pay scrupulous attention to personal hygiene.

● Always wipe from front to back after opening your bowels, to prevent contamination of the vagina with bacteria from the anus.

● Go for cotton underwear and avoid tight jeans and knickers.

● If you have a new sexual partner, or you think your regular sex partner could have an infection, always use a condom.

● A cupful of vinegar in the bath water occasionally can

---

help the vagina maintain its acid balance, which may prevent infection taking hold.

- Avoid using flannels and sponges to wash your genitals, as they can harbour infection – and never use flannels, sponges or towels belonging to anyone else for cleaning or drying this intimate area.
- Be on the lookout for any signs and symptoms of vaginal infection, such as unusual vaginal discharge, one which is more smelly or profuse than usual, itching, or soreness and consult your doctor or visit the GU clinic without delay.
- Go for regular check-ups at the GU clinic, especially if you change your partner.
- Make sure your partner keeps his penis and beneath his foreskin clean.
- If you undergo any gynaecological procedures such as abortion, having an IUD fitted, D & C, fetal monitoring and so on, ideally you should ask to be tested for disease-causing organisms before you undergo the procedures. In practice this isn't very often possible. However, you should insist on being tested if you have any suspicious symptoms.
- If you have to have any gynaecological procedures, be on the lookout for signs of infection or vague feelings of illness afterwards and get a check-up.

Chapter 5

Diagnostic Dilemmas

If you have any of the symptoms of PID it's vital to get a diagnosis and begin treatment as soon as possible. With proper early treatment, PID is curable and you can avoid the months of pain, exhaustion and strain on a partnership, not to mention the long-term complications.

It's important to avoid even a short delay in getting treatment: one researcher found that the majority of women treated within two days recovered totally, while those in whom treatment was delayed by as little as a week faced more serious consequences. Treatment that is delayed for any reason is also less effective, because by then the damage may have already been done. Some doctors believe swift, accurate diagnosis and treatment of PID could cut female infertility by a tenth.

It sounds simple enough, but getting treatment can be easier said than done. British genito-urinary specialist Dr Patricia Munday has said, 'Diagnosis is the crux of the (PID) problem.' Yet countless PID sufferers have discovered to their bitter cost that their symptoms are often underplayed. Even when they are recognized, they may be dismissed as being of no importance. This attitude seems especially blinkered when you consider the potentially devastating consequences of the illness.

Libby's Story

'It started when I noticed I was having to get up to pass water during the night. At the same time I had a constant ache in my pelvis. My GP referred me to a urologist, who took samples and said I needed a bladder stretch, to enable it to hold more water. However, that didn't work and I continued to get problems. After about a year of being under the urologist they decided that maybe the problems were gynaecological. I'd had a long-term history of thrush, so although I had a vaginal discharge that was normal for me and I didn't think anything of it. The gynaecologist said it wasn't normal, though. He treated me with pessaries and then discharged me. However, the problems continued, and eventually the gynaecologist diagnosed irritable bowel syndrome and told me to eat more fibre. I continued to get the pain, and eventually went back to the urologist who examined me and looked at my cervix. She discovered a terrible purulent discharge which filled half a test tube. She sent that to be tested and cauterized my cervix. But to her amazement, when the results came back they were negative. She did another cauterization and prescribed more drugs. The fourth time I went, I saw another doctor who diagnosed a cyst on my ovary, which I had to have removed. Afterwards they told me the cyst had burst and oozed out all over the pelvic cavity, so they had to do a big clean-up job. Six weeks later I was in agony, all on my right side. I couldn't stand up to iron, or carry heavy shopping. After that I got fed up with all the toing and froing so I plodded on for a bit. But eventually I was having to miss so much work that I decided to pay privately to have a laparoscopy. They discovered I had massive adhesions that had caused my womb to stick to the front of my pelvis. But, amazingly, when they did a test for chlamydia it came back clear. I couldn't believe it.'

Barriers To Diagnosis

The founder of the British PID Support Network, Jessica Pickard, was herself a sufferer. She lists several reasons why so many sufferers find it difficult to get an accurate diagnosis, which include:

- PID is a disease affecting only women, and even today most doctors are mainly men.

- Pain is a 'normal' experience for women – for example, period pains, childbirth pains and so on – so complaints of pain from a woman are more likely to be ignored or dismissed as 'part of being a woman'. One researcher found that almost half of women who were told they didn't have PID did in fact have the illness.

- Women's complaints are more likely to be dismissed as trivial, especially where tests show no physical reason for symptoms, so the necessary follow-up tests or further investigations may never be carried out.

- PID has a low profile medically. It is not a glamorous topic for medical research and so it doesn't attract funding. Because it can be chronic there is less likelihood of a 'miracle cure' being found.

- Because PID is linked to female sexuality, many doctors are uncomfortable with it, as is society generally. The infections that can lead on to PID are often equated with promiscuity.

Between Two Stools

There are other reasons why PID may not be adequately diagnosed.

One of the main problems is that it doesn't fit neatly into any one medical speciality. As Libby's story so neatly illustrates, sufferers may be seen by any one of a host of different specialists. By the time you get a diagnosis it's not uncommon for sufferers to have see the GP, a general surgeon, a urologist, a genito-urinary physician, or a gynaecologist. It may be many years after the vague vaginal infection you had in your teens or early twenties when you reach the infertility clinic and it is found you have blocked tubes. By that time you may even have forgotten about the original episode.

Another factor is that the symptoms may be mild, vague and easily confused with other illnesses. They may clear up, or appear to clear up of their own accord, when in fact what has happened is that the disease has spread up to the reproductive organs where it continues to wreak its silent damage.

Separating PID From Other Pelvic Problems

To complicate matters even further, PID is incredibly difficult to diagnose accurately. Gynaecologist Malcolm Pearce of St George's Hospital, London, writing in the *British Medical Journal* in 1990 says, 'It is usually badly managed by doctors with little interest in the condition.'

The only certain way to detect PID is to carry out a laparoscopy – an operation in which the doctor examines the reproductive organs using a special micro-telescope. One now-famous study carried out in Sweden in the 1960s found that of 800 women confidently diagnosed as having pelvic infection by experienced gynaecologists, only just over 60 per cent were found to actually have PID when they underwent laparoscopy. The other 30-odd per cent had a variety of other problems, some trivial, some serious and in some cases no diagnosis could be reached. 'All too often the diagnosis tends to be a dustbin for all sorts of non-specific lower abdominal pain in young women,' says Pearce. That means that a staggering 35 out of every 100 women with quite severe signs and symptoms of the disease actually did not have it. At the same time the same researchers carried out laparoscopy on a large number of other women who had provisional diagnoses of some other condition. To their surprise a considerable number of these actually had PID. So there are errors on both sides. The results of this, and several other studies which have replicated it, make it clear that accurate diagnosis of PID is abysmal.

Overdiagnosis and Underdiagnosis

The reason for such mistakes lies in the way PID is traditionally diagnosed. You go to the doctor complaining of pelvic pain. He or she palpates your abdomen to see if it feels tender, and asks you about any symptoms. For most women, pelvic pain is the main physical sign. On the other hand, pelvic pain can also be an indicator of other conditions.

Many doctors – and unfortunately, gynaecologists tend be particular culprits in this respect – believe that if you have pain and tenderness you have PID, and that if you have pain but no tenderness you haven't. The Swedish study showed that the question was much more complex than that, but it didn't filter through to many gynaecologists.

Just to complicate matters still further, the message *did* get through to genito-urinary specialists, with the result that almost every woman who walked through the door of the GU clinic complaining of pelvic pain would automatically be dished out antibiotics, without further investigations being carried out. And while this may have benefited some women with pelvic pain, many others would return for repeated rounds of antibiotics until finally they were labelled as having chronic PID without having had a proper diagnosis in the first place.

Another study of 150 women with pelvic pain who had laparoscopies carried out in the GU clinic at St Mary's Hospital, London, showed that only one in five had PID, and the other four had other diagnoses. It's clear that your diagnosis could well depend on who you see. PID tends to be over-diagnosed by GU specialists, whereas it is underdiagnosed by gynaecologists. Somewhere in between we have GPs who may or may not refer you on for further specialist investigations, but who may not have adequate testing facilities for diagnosis.

The Case for Laparoscopy

The only certain way to diagnose PID is to have a laparoscopy, in which the doctor examines your reproductive organs by means of a special microscope inserted through the abdominal wall. Gynaecologist John Hare says, 'Where laparoscopy has been used accuracy [of diagnosis] is around 95 per cent, which is a great improvement on the usual figure of 65 per cent, even in good units.'

In an ideal world, many doctors believe, all women with suspected PID should have a laparoscopy. Not only would this improve diagnosis by enabling the doctor to exclude other pelvic problems, it would also make it possible to collect specimens of fluid to be tested for infectious organisms from the reproductive organs. Such specimens are known to be more reliable than those taken from the cervix, since the tubes are the most frequent site of infection, and cervical antibodies can neutralize infection.

However, most specialists say it would be impracticable and expensive to carry out a laparoscopy for all suspected cases of PID. As Malcolm Pearce points out in his *BMJ* article on PID: 'Diagnostic laparoscopy seems unacceptable to most gynaecologists . . .despite the low risk of complications from the procedure.'

Instead, treatment tends to be a matter of trial and error. You will be doled out antibiotics. You will be offered laparoscopy only if you don't respond to antibiotic treatment, or if the doctor can detect a definite swelling or 'mass', which could indicate an abscess, when he or she palpates your abdomen.

Unfortunately, as Pearce points out, 'This policy makes little sense, for only 32 per cent of clinical masses are confirmed at laparoscopy, and 9 per cent of masses seen at laparoscopy are not clinically apparent.'

One of the problems, as John Hare points out, is that GU physicians see so many cases of vaginal infection, yet they don't have access to laparoscopic testing, which is the preserve of gynaecologists.

Practicalities

So where does that leave you if you have symptoms of PID? The first step is usually to consult your GP. In this case you may be treated straight away with a short course of antibiotics.

However, it may be a better bet to head straight for the GU clinic, where the doctors have the expertise and facilities for more accurate diagnosis. In the UK, changes in GPs' contracts introduced in 1990 have meant that many more are offering diagnostic tests of various kinds. Many GPs, though, still lack the skills or time to cope with problems like PID. It's not a good idea to keep messing about with different antibiotics and hoping for the best.

Make a list of your symptoms and keep a note of when they first occurred, what if anything may have sparked them off and what makes them better or worse. Be prepared to be persistent. Doctors are slowly becoming more knowledgeable about PID, thanks to the efforts of organizations such as the PID Support Network, but there are still those who are ignorant, or who may attempt to fob you off. If you have visited a GP and PID is suspected, he or she may refer you to a gynaecologist or GU specialist for further tests and treatment.

You And Your Doctor

If you feel that you aren't being helped by your doctor, then you can ask to be referred for a second opinion. This could either be with another doctor in the practice, a doctor whom you trust in another practice, a specialist such as a gynaecologist or a genito-urinary physician. If you really feel you aren't getting a proper diagnosis, the PID Support Network can help put you in touch with a sympathetic and knowledgeable doctor, NHS or private (if you can afford it) through their contacts throughout the UK.

What Will The Doctor Do?

Take A Case History

He or she should ask you about your symptoms, when you first noticed them, how severe they are, and what if anything makes them better or worse.

Take Your Temperature

If you have an acute attack of PID, a temperature of over 38°C (100.4°F) in combination with other signs and symptoms could suggest PID.

Pelvic Examination

The doctor should then gently palpate your abdomen to see whether it is painful, and try and detect the source of the pain. In addition, s/he may also do an internal examination. Two fingers are inserted into your vagina while the doctor feels your abdomen with the other hand to try and locate any tenderness and swelling.

The doctor might then examine your cervix using a speculum. She or he will move your cervix around to see whether motion causes pain, and will look for any signs of discharge or pus.

Take Swabs

The doctor should then take one or several swabs of mucus from your cervix. In a GU clinic, these can be examined immediately for pus and the bacteria that cause gonorrhoea, and other swabs can be sent for culturing. The doctor will also want to look for chlamydia, and other organisms that might be causing the problem. The doctor should also take swabs from the urethra (the passage that leads from the bladder), and may occasionally take a swab from the anus.

These tests are important because they help the doctor to identify the precise bacteria which are causing the problems, and therefore choose the most appropriate treatment. However, as we saw in previous chapters, the swabs may not always show signs of infection, since infection may already have moved up from the cervix into the tubes.

Checking Your Partner

As we have seen, the organisms causing PID are often silent, and recurrences can happen as a result of re-infection. Partners of women with non-specific PID (where the cause cannot be isolated) have been shown to have gonorrhoea in about 15 per cent of cases, and be infected with chlamydia in 12 per cent of cases. It is therefore vital that your partner is tested and treated too.

Although this is standard practice in GU clinics, it may not be done if you are seen by your GP or a gynaecologist. If it is not offered, it is worth asking your doctor if this can be done, and if you are met with a refusal, encourage your partner to attend the GU clinic. Do bear in mind too that your partner could re-infect you without having any actual symptoms himself, and insist that he attends for a test.

Blood and Urine Tests

Blood tests may be carried out to see whether your levels of white blood cells are raised. If they are, it can be sign that infection is present, and your body is trying to fight it. You can, of course, have PID and have normal blood cell levels, so such tests are only useful if carried out in conjunction with the other tests mentioned. Blood and urine tests should also be carried out to exclude other sexually transmitted disease. Women with PID also have higher levels of certain chemical markers in the blood, and these can be used to detect the severity of the condition.

Ultrasound

An ultrasound scan to examine your reproductive organs may be performed. This may be more likely to be done if you are seen by a gynaecologist rather than a GU specialist. The scanner works by bouncing sound waves off a solid object to produce a picture of your pelvic organs. It can show up any areas of swelling or pus, but it is not always accurate. The scan may be performed abdominally, in which case a special gel which helps create a better picture is smoothed over your abdomen. Then a hand-held transducer – a device that picks up sound signals and transforms them into a pictorial form that can be viewed on the screen – is passed slowly over your abdomen and the picture appears on the screen. In a vaginal scan, the transducer takes the form of a long thin instrument a bit like a pen. The doctor gently inserts it into your vagina and the resulting picture appears on the screen.

Endometrial Biopsy

This is a procedure which is used far more in Scandinavia and the USA for diagnosing PID. It involves passing a fine tube into the uterus with a sharp cutting edge, or applying suction to take a small sample of tissue from the womb lining (endometrium).

The operation can be performed without an anaesthetic and although most women spend a day in hospital, it can be done on an outpatient basis. Results are usually available within two to three days, and recent studies have shown it to be remarkably accurate. One Finnish expert writing recently says, 'Endometrial biopsy should be used more often among patients with suspected PID.'

Laparoscopy

Although many doctors feel this should be done as routine, in practice it is only likely to be performed if clinical examination is not conclusive or if antibiotic treatment doesn't help. It involves puncturing a small hole in your abdomen, just below the navel. Carbon dioxide is used to inflate the abdomen, and a special microscope with a light on the end is inserted. Another tiny hole is made on the 'bikini line' so that the doctor can insert a probe enabling him or her to move the pelvic organs around in order to examine them. The doctor can see whether there is any redness or swelling and can detect any other pelvic problems such as scarring or an ovarian abscess which may be causing symptoms. He or she can also take fluid samples for bacteriological testing.

What Else Could It Be?

There are many other causes of pelvic pain besides PID, and the doctor needs to rule these out before concluding that your symptoms are caused by PID. However, in view of the fact that PID can have such terrible consequences, many doctors believe it is better to overtreat a case of potential infection than to miss an acute case of PID, however mild the symptoms.

Other problems include:

- **Pelvic adhesions**: scar tissue caused by previous infections or surgery.

- **Endometriosis**: when parts of the lining of the uterus (the endometrium) migrate to other areas of the pelvic cavity. The tissue continues to respond to the female hormones by menstruating, but because there is nowhere for the blood to go it collects and forms painful scar tissue.

- **Ovarian problems**: for example, a ruptured ovarian cyst, polycystic ovaries, in which tiny cysts grow on the ovaries, or an ovarian tumour. An ultrasound scan would show whether any of these were the problem.

- **Fibroids**: more common in women over 35, and they rarely cause pain, but nevertheless a possibility.

- **Ectopic pregnancy:** in which the unborn baby begins to develop in the fallopian tubes. This often happens because of damage or blockage to the tubes, which is frequently caused by PID. Sadly, pregnancy cannot continue in this case. The condition can result in a painful and dangerous miscarriage. An ultrasound scan is used to diagnose the condition, and the affected fallopian tube usually has to be removed.

- **Acute appendicitis.**

- **Sexual abuse**: it's been discovered that in many cases of pelvic pain where no signs of PID can be detected, the woman has been sexually abused as a child. That's not to say that women who have been sexually abused cannot also have real PID. Women who have been sexually abused often find any kind of gynaecological investigation extremely traumatic. However, if this applies to you, it is particularly important to get a proper diagnosis, so you can get the help and counselling you almost certainly need.

- **Irritable bowel syndrome (spastic colon):** in a study of 55 women, aged between 18 and 35, with pelvic pain, 30 had symptoms of irritable bowel syndrome. Other symptoms include pain that gets better when you open your bowels, loose bowel motions when the pain starts, more frequent bowel motions when pain starts, pelletty stools, alternating diarrhoea and constipation, incomplete emptying of the bowels and passing mucus in the motions. Conventional treatment involves reassurance that nothing serious is wrong, increasing the amount of fibre consumed, and in some more severe cases, sedatives to calm the bowel or drugs to control symptoms of diarrhoea and constipation. Alternative therapies which have proved helpful include stress-reduction techniques, hypnotherapy, acupuncture, homoeopathy and herbal treatment.

If you discover any blood in your bowel motions you should always consult a doctor.

Pelvic congestion

One of the most important conditions that has until recently often been confused with PID is pelvic congestion. Until the last few years, doctors often argued that the condition – caused by enlarged veins in the uterus – was a myth, and dismissed women suffering chronic pelvic pain as neurotic. However, pioneering research carried out at St Mary's Hospital, London, using a special sort of vein x-ray, has shown that the condition exists. In fact, more than eight out of ten women complaining of pelvic pain for which no cause can be found on laparoscopy are found to have enlarged veins in the uterus. The veins are often three times their normal diameter.

The pain, usually a dull ache, gets worse with standing or exercise and better with rest. Pelvic congestion also causes painful periods, bleeding irregularities and pain during sex or at orgasm. What happens is that when the veins become enlarged, they cause the blood to stagnate and slow circulation in the pelvic area.

The condition is thought to be linked to an excess of the female sex hormone oestrogen, produced by the ovaries. Alternatively it could be that women suffering pelvic congestion are for some reason reacting to normal oestrogen levels. This has been confirmed by research in which ultrasound scans of women with chronic pelvic pain due to pelvic congestion. They were found to have other changes in the uterus and ovaries suggestive of increased concentrations of or hypersensitivity to oestrogen.

Treatment is with a drug such as dihydroergotamine, which narrows the veins, given by injection during an acute attack. Alternatively a drug called medroxyprogesterone acetate, which quells the activity of the ovaries, or a certain type of hormone replacement therapy, may be used.

Being Taken Seriously

One of the biggest problems for women suffering pelvic pain of any origin, according to the Canadian PID Society, is convincing doctors that the pain is a symptom of a physical problem. In this case they advise getting a second opinion. In the meantime you should rest, abstain from lovemaking, and eat light nutritious meals.

Because PID can so often mimic or be confused with other conditions, if your symptoms don't respond to treatment you should ask for further investigations to be carried out. However, do bear in mind that once PID has set in it may

take a long time to clear up. In other cases the damage which
has already been done can create further problems, such as
pain caused by scarring.

Chapter 6

Fighting PID – The Orthodox Way

PID is a serious illness, and serious illnesses call for serious measures. It's universally agreed that antibiotics are vital to knock any infection on the head. However, that's about as far as the agreement goes. One of the big problems with PID is that doctors still can't agree among themselves on the best antibiotics to use, how often they should be taken or the length of time treatment should continue.

Once treatment is started, the bacteria should be killed off and symptoms disappear quickly. Acute, subclinical or recurrent PID seem to respond best to antibiotics. Chronic PID is more difficult to treat, because many doctors believe that symptoms are caused not by active infection, but by the results of infection. Some doctors still believe that antibiotics have a useful part to play in knocking out any lingering pockets of infection, but many women themselves feel their problems are just made worse by taking constant courses of antibiotics.

Doctors are still arguing about whether PID is caused by one single organism or by several. The latest thinking veers towards the view that an initial infection with gonorrhoea, chlamydia or both allows other aerobic and anaerobic bacteria to take hold. In order to knock out all possible organisms, a cocktail of different antibiotics is often used. The trouble is that mixing antibiotics in this way increases the risk of side-effects, and with it the risk that you are less likely to continue treatment. Alternatively, the doctor may decide to use what is known as a broad spectrum antibiotic – one that is effective against a wide range of different bacteria.

Doctors are still trying to work out the most effective combinations of drugs and length of treatment. It is thought that too long courses of antibiotics – more than three weeks – can actually be detrimental, by lowering the body's resistance to infection, and may lead to the more rapid development of antibiotic-resistant strains of bacteria, making the illness yet more difficult to treat in the future.

Emergency!

Emergency surgery is essential if you have a burst abscess, or if the doctor thinks any abscesses are likely to rupture. Unless an operation is performed right away peritonitis – inflammation of the pelvic cavity – could ensue, with possibly fatal results. Unfortunately, some doctors can be a bit too casual about removing body parts while they are at it: it is not unknown for women to wake up after such surgery to find their uterus and/or ovaries have been removed. Once this has been done you can wave goodbye to any chances of having a baby. Of course it may be necessary if the organs are found to be badly affected or damaged, and in a real emergency there may be no time to make choices. However, if there is time beforehand you should ask the doctor exactly what he is planning to do. No one can operate on you until you have signed the consent form, and it is possible to amend the form to include your wishes.

Home Or Hospital?

Many experts believe that all victims of acute PID should be admitted to hospital for a day or so. The arguments in favour of this are that there are facilities for instant diagnosis and monitoring, and treatment can be given direct into the bloodstream by means of intravenous drugs – faster and more effective than taking drugs by mouth. On the other hand, going into hospital upsets your life.

American PID expert Dr David Hemsell, writing in the *Journal of Reproductive Medicine* in 1988, recommends hospital admission in all the following cases:

- those where diagnosis is uncertain
- those with an inflammation and swelling or where an abscess is known to be present or suspected
- anyone who is pregnant. The illness can be extremely dangerous for both mothers-to-be and their babies and immediate treatment is vital
- pre-teenage children (PID is very rare in this group except in those who have been sexually abused)
- anyone who is severely ill with an attack, or where it is suspected the attack has spread to the ovaries, tubes or pelvic cavity
- those who can't tolerate treatment or are unable to follow it properly because of side-effects, nausea, vomiting, pain or other reasons
- those who are not cured by initial treatment or who cannot be checked by a doctor two or three days after such treatment
- women who have never had a baby and wish to do so, and those who haven't yet completed their families.

In Britain, women with PID are usually admitted to hospital only if the infection is suspected to have spread to the tubes or ovaries, or if the doctor can feel a definite swelling in the abdomen.

What Drugs Will Be Given?

It's important that you are prescribed the right antibiotics. Penicillins and a type of drug called cephalosporins are ineffective against the major causes of PID. However, they are still widely prescribed in the mistaken belief that most PID arises from infection with gonorrhoea.

Where symptoms suggest only mild PID, it may be decided to treat you with co-trimoxazole, which is effective against a wide range of infective agents, and metronidazole (Flagyl). Drugs of the tetracycline group of antibiotics, such as doxycycline, (or erythromycin if you are pregnant) will also be prescribed. They are effective against over 90 per cent of the organisms known to cause PID. The doctor will want to check up on you in two or three days' time. And if there are no signs of definite improvement, in an ideal world you should be admitted to hospital for a laparoscopy to try and track down the exact source of the trouble. If results of the swabs show a specific organism to be the cause of your symptoms, the doctor may alter the prescription during treatment to an agent known to be active against that particular organism. Of course, we don't live in an ideal world, and what tends to happen in practice is that you are prescribed different antibiotics in an ever-more-frantic hit and miss search for the cause of the problems. It may be worth asking your doctor if you can be referred for laparoscopy if symptoms don't appear to be clearing within three days.

Current recommendations for more severe acute PID include a single dose of ampicillin and probenecid, effective against gonorrhoea. This may be followed by a week of treatment with a strong broad spectrum antibiotic such as gentamicyn or tobramycin, effective against certain organisms known to cause PID, and metronidazole (Flagyl), which is effective against anaerobic bacteria, for two weeks.

In addition, doctors recommend at least a two-week follow-up course of doxycycline or erythromycin to wipe out any last traces of chlamydia.

Keep Taking the Tablets

It's vital that you should take the treatment exactly as it is prescribed. Make sure you take the whole course of treatment. Don't stop taking the tablets just because you feel better, since this could lead to the infection not being properly wiped out and the development of antibiotic-resistant organisms which are harder to treat effectively.

In the past, it was customary to prescribe short courses of tetracyclines – say up to ten days – which are sufficient to clear chlamydia from the cervix. However, it is now realized that this may not be adequate to eradicate the infection from the upper genital tract, where infection can persist and cause irreversible tissue damage.

Before taking the treatment, tell your doctor about any other medication you may be taking (including the contraceptive pill), any other illnesses you might have such as kidney problems, and if you think you might be pregnant, since certain drugs or combinations might be contraindicated.

Side-effects

The powerful antibiotics used to treat PID may in themselves bring on unpleasant side-effects. Flagyl, for example, can cause nausea, vomiting, stomach upsets and diarrhoea. You should avoid drinking alcohol if you are taking it, as the two react with each other to accentuate the effects of both.

Thrush, caused by the yeast *Candida albicans*, is a common side-effect of antibiotics. It happens because the antibiotics wipe out not just the bacteria which are causing infection, but also other bacteria which normally keep the yeast in check. Treatment consists either of a single tablet of an anti-thrush drug, such as Canestan, or nystatin pessaries, which you insert into your vagina. Nystatin can also be prescribed to be taken by mouth for severe cases of thrush, but that in turn can make you feel nauseous. Many women find that eating live yogurt or taking acidophilus tablets (available from the health food shop or chemist), which help restore the balance of bacteria, can help protect against thrush.

Because antibiotics are so powerful they can make you feel run down generally, so it is wise to look after yourself while you are taking them. Make sure you eat a good, varied diet, with plenty of fresh fruit and vegetables. Get plenty of rest and sleep too (see Bedrest below).

Jane's Story

'I developed PID following a caesarean section in which my bladder was ruptured. The first attack I had, I ended up in hospital, where I was put on intravenous antibiotics. Things started to clear up after that but for the next three years I was plagued by lower pelvic pain. I also kept getting cystitis. Eventually I was referred to a urologist, who wanted to stretch my urethra. I refused to have that done, because I thought the scarring would just make things worse. The doctor put me on several courses of antibiotics, but I got very run down with all that medication, and I was in constant pain. Eventually I decided to come off the antibiotics because they didn't seem to be making things any better, and I felt lousy all the time. I visited a naturopath who put me on a detoxifying diet, because I was so full of antibiotics that my immune system was low. I also took a course of lactobacillus [acidophilus] tablets, and at last I began to feel better than I had done for ages.'

PID and Your Partner

It's vital that any sex partner you have should also be treated in order to avoid re-infection. With each recurrent attack of PID, the more difficult it is to treat, and the greater the chances of severe long-term problems. If your doctor doesn't offer to do this, you should insist that your partner visits the GU clinic. Even if your partner has no symptoms, he could be a silent carrier of infection. If you know or suspect that your partner may have sex with other people besides you, it is vital they are treated too. One of the biggest problems of breaking the chain of infection that leads to PID, according to John Hare, is that many GU clinics don't carry out automatic 'contact tracing' for chlamydia.

He says 'In Sweden, where chlamydia is covered by STD regulation, contact tracing for male infections is a legal requirement. The most useful way forward in this country would be for contact tracing to be carried out. GPs should be discouraged from treating male cases of urethritis, which should be treated by GU physicians.'

If you are asked to give the name of your sex partner, when you visit the clinic, it's important not to be evasive. You can rest assured that any contact tracing that is carried out will be discreet and that your partner and/or his partners will not need to know that you are involved, unless you choose to tell them. However, if you are being treated by a GP or gynaecologist, this service may not be offered.

It's important to refrain from making love until you receive the all-clear and you know for certain that both you and your partner are free from infection. The thrusting actions of sex moves the pelvic organs and can spread pus and infection through the tubes and into the pelvic cavity.

Follow-up

It's vital to attend for a follow-up check once you have

finished antibiotic treatment. Chlamydia in particular has a nasty habit of coming back again. One study showed a third of men treated for chlamydia had recurrences despite treatment – and half of these repeated infections occurred more than two weeks after treatment was completed. Some experts believe you should attend for repeated check-ups for a year after treatment to make sure any infection is completely wiped out.

For the same reason it's important to let the doctor know if you still feel ill despite treatment. There have been cases where women have been pronounced cured despite the fact that they felt unwell, and who subsequently went on to develop long-term health problems. If your doctor doesn't take you seriously, seek a second opinion.

If treatment fails, however, you should avoid taking repeated courses of different antibiotics. These can wear down the body's own natural defence system, laying it open to further infections. It's vital to not to get into a vicious circle of infection and treatment, followed by repeated infection. You must have further investigations to sort out the roots of the problem.

Bedrest

It may be tempting to struggle on, especially if your symptoms are mild, or if you have a busy job or young children to cope with. However, the experts are agreed that bedrest is absolutely vital to prevent infection from spreading and to allow your body time to heal. Not all doctors recognize the importance of rest, but the various PID support groups believe it is essential if proper healing is to take place.

The Canadian PID Society warn in their leaflet, 'The correct antibiotic may not cure PID without this rest,' and add, 'A woman who has PID should stay in bed until at least two days after her temperature is normal and there is no pain.'

Once you do start to feel better, take it easy, and don't rush back into your normal activities until you get the all-clear from the doctor. It can take between two and six weeks before you are able to be properly up and about again. However, it is important. In the British Women's Reproductive Rights Information Centre's leaflet on PID, they cite the case of a woman who followed her doctor's orders to stay in bed for six weeks during an attack of PID and completely recovered. When, a few years later, she developed a second attack, and a different doctor advised her to resume her normal activities, the PID got worse and continues to plague her even today.

The WRRIC leaflet goes on to say: 'Many women are used to dragging themselves through illnesses for the sake of family or work, but with PID you should not be tempted to do this. If your infection is not defeated in its early phase, there is a danger that you may become very ill indeed. It's a false calculation to struggle on, because in the long run you won't be able to keep up your commitment to other people, and . . . you are endangering your own long term health.'

Life From The Bedside

Bedrest is only effective if you rest completely. Here are a few ideas to help you do so:

● Get someone to buy you in food that is easy to eat and needs no preparation. Keep a selection covered on a tray or trolley next to the bed, so you don't have to bother with preparing yourself meals. Ideas include hard boiled eggs, stuffed eggs, cocktail sausages, meatballs, or vegetarian nut balls or burgers, sandwiches, and a selection of fruit, nuts, and vegetables such as carrot sticks, celery, baby tomatoes and so on. Keep a knife, tin opener, and rubbish bag within easy reach too. In the winter you might include a wide-necked thermos of soup or a casserole.

- Keep a kettle or teasmade together with tea and coffee, dried milk, or a selection of herbal teabags next to the bed.

- A neighbour or friend might be willing to bring you a portion of whatever she is preparing for her family.

- Get your partner to stop off at the local deli or takeaway on the way back from work occasionally.

- Enlist the help of friends. Get one friend to organize a rota of people who can come in and do odd jobs for you such as washing up, doing the laundry, ironing, cleaning and so on.

- Your GP, health visitor or a social worker may be able to arrange for you to have temporary home help or meals on wheels until you feel better.

- If possible, have a phone point installed in your bedroom, and keep the phone within easy reach. Contact with the outside world is important while you are bedridden.

- Keep other useful things such as writing paper, books, sewing things or anything else you might need in a cupboard next to your bed.

- If you can afford it, consider investing in a portable TV, preferably with a remote control, to keep in the bedroom. Alternatively, keep a portable radio at your bedside.

- Invest in one of those special trays on a trolley that fits over the bed. Organizations such as Disabled Living Foundation (380-384 Harrow Road, London N9 2HU) may have other practical suggestions that can help make life easier while you are confined to the bedroom.

The Next Step – Surgery?

If antibiotics don't clear up symptoms, it could be that irreversible damage has already been done to the pelvic organs. In this case you have two choices: to learn to live with your symptoms (see Chapter 8, Living With PID) or to opt for surgery. Such operations are called elective – or planned – surgery. It is worth thinking very carefully if surgery is suggested, since even though such surgery can remove lingering pockets of infection, many PID sufferers continue to experience persistent pain afterwards.

What Might Be Done?

● Removal of thickened and scar tissue. So long as no active infection is present, surgery can be carried out to remove scar tissue (adhesions), which may be hampering free movement of the pelvic organs and causing pain. Using sophisticated techniques of microsurgery, the surgeon is able, during a laparoscopy (see page 64), to separate any organs that have stuck together. Alternatively a laparotomy, which involves making a slightly larger incision, may be carried out. However, this in itself can sometimes create yet more scar tissue, so compounding the original problem.

● Removal of the fallopian tubes (salpingectomy). Where infection of the tubes has become chronic, the surgeon may suggest removing of all or part of the tubes. Such surgery is difficult to carry out technically, and even with surgery symptoms may persist. The operation may also cause scar tissue to form, and will mean that natural conception is no longer possible. If you want a baby you will have to opt for one of the assisted conception techniques such as IVF (in vitro fertilization or 'test tube baby').

● Hysterectomy (removal of the womb). This is a major operation, and you need to consider it carefully and make sure that you are certain that all other avenues have been explored before going ahead. The operation can take six months or longer to recover from. Having a hysterectomy will also mean coming to terms with the end of your fertility; since women's reproductive abilities are so closely tied with their sexuality, some women see themselves as less feminine and desirable after a hysterectomy. If the surgery works, others are so grateful to be free of pain and other problems that they feel a renewed sense of zest and well-being or energy.

As with any pelvic surgery, scar tissue can form and cause problems. What is more, there is no guarantee that pelvic pain will go once you have had the operation, and the operation itself can have side-effects. However, many women who have been plagued with recurrent pelvic problems report a new lease of life once they have had a hysterectomy.

Hysterectomy is sometimes combined with removal of the ovaries (oophorectomy). If this is done you will be thrown into the menopause, and could be faced with a whole new set of health problems. Premature menopause brought on by surgery is known to create more severe menopausal symptoms (such as hot flushes, night sweats, vaginal dryness, sexual problems, and depression) than menopause that takes place naturally. The risk of problems – such as osteoporosis and heart disease – which affect women after the menopause is also increased after a premature menopause. To prevent these, doctors usually suggest hormone replacement therapy (HRT).

● Presacral neurectomy. This is an operation in which the presacral nerve, which serves the pelvic area, is removed. The operation is tricky to perform, since the nerve runs close to large blood vessels. The operation is very rarely performed in the UK. However, in the US, where the operation is more common, it is claimed to be 75 per cent effective in getting rid of pelvic pain. The operation will only be considered when active infection is not present, since otherwise all it would do is remove the symptoms of trouble rather than tackling the underlying cause. There may be temporary loss of bowel and bladder control.

Chapter 7

PID And Your Fertility

One in six couples face problems conceiving, and blocked tubes comes second only to ovulation problems in the list of causes. Chlamydial PID – when scar tissues blocks the tubes wholly or partially – is the most preventable cause of blocked tubes. Even if you do manage to conceive, PID and chlamydia can cause problems. PID is responsible for ectopic (or tubal pregnancy) when the unborn baby grows outside the uterus, usually in the fallopian tube, and chlamydia is thought to be the culprit in some cases of miscarriage and perinatal death.

Ectopic Pregnancy

Linda's Story

'I was on the Pill for ten years when my GP suggested coming off it. At that time I was sleeping with one person on a regular basis, but he wasn't my only sexual partner and nor was I his. The doctor and I talked about other methods of contraception and she suggested the IUD. She warned me of the risk of infection, but I decided to go ahead. Within a month of having the IUD fitted I developed a severe vaginal infection. I was given antibiotics but they didn't work. I continued to have symptoms and I also had shooting pains in my vagina. I went to see the doctor again who did an internal and took some swabs. She said the infection had got to my ovaries and gave me some more antibiotics, but it still didn't go away. Eventually they removed the IUD and treated me with Flagyl which cleared up the infection and I didn't think anything more about it. However, four years ago I became pregnant. I had five negative pregnancy tests, so finally I went to the Pregnancy Advisory Service who did a blood test and confirmed that I was pregnant. Later that day I started to bleed and the doctor said she thought I was miscarrying. She sent me to the hospital for a scan where they told me they couldn't see anything in my uterus and told me to come back the next day for a laparoscopy. I went to see a friend, and while I was there I collapsed in terrible pain, with what I now recognize were the symptoms of shock. I was shaking and had cold sweats and was feeling very odd. I wanted to go home to bed, but I didn't have the money for a taxi and I felt too ill to go by public transport. Eventually we went to the outpatient department of the hospital where I collapsed. They took me into a side ward and asked 'Is there anything we should know?' As it happened I had a letter in my bag from the ultrasound department which said 'suspected ectopic pregnancy'. They operated immediately. When I came to they told me the tube had completely ruptured and that I had haemorrhaged badly into my stomach. They hadn't been able to save the ovary or fallopian tube. I asked what caused it, and they said they didn't know. It was only quite a while later that I began to think that the severe infection I had all those years ago could have been the cause.'

As Linda's story shows, an ectopic pregnancy is a traumatic and distressing experience. One in every 200 pregnancies is ectopic, and the condition is on the increase. According to one doctor who has specialized in the subject, a dramatic rise in the incidence of diagnosed ectopic pregnancy has been reported at an annual increase of 4.8 per cent in England and Wales, 6.3 per cent in Canada and 8.6 per cent in California.

It is no coincidence that the dramatic upturn in ectopic pregnancy has gone hand in hand with the rise in PID and chlamydia. The good news is that better diagnostic methods such as vaginal ultrasound scanning and the existence of ultra-sensitive pregnancy tests mean that such pregnancies can now be picked up early, before the tube bursts as it did in Linda's case.

Why It Happens

Normally when you become pregnant an egg is released from the ovary into the fallopian tube where it is fertilized by sperm. Once sperm and egg have fused they spend the next three days being wafted down the fallopian tube to the womb. If, however, the fallopian tube is blocked because of scar tissue, the embryo gets stuck and continues to grow in the tube.

In many cases the embryo dies and is reabsorbed by the body. If this happens, apart from your period being a few days late you may never be aware that you have conceived. However, if the embryo continues to grow it gradually stretches the tube; such a pregnancy cannot survive for longer than twelve to fourteen weeks at the most because the embryo becomes so large that the tube bursts. Severe pain and bleeding set in, with sometimes fatal results. This is a life-threatening emergency, as shock can set in and there is a very real danger of bleeding to death. It is vital to get the condition diagnosed as quickly as possible so that the pregnancy can be terminated. In the past this used to mean surgery to remove the affected fallopian tube, but today new techniques of surgery and non-surgical methods are becoming an option.

Symptoms

Sufferers experience all the normal symptoms of early pregnancy such as nausea, vomiting, tender breasts, and lack of periods. However, because there are lower levels of hormones in an ectopic pregnancy, sufferers may not experience symptoms such as morning sickness so strongly. The abdomen starts to swell just as if the baby had implanted in the uterus. A clue that the pregnancy may be ectopic is if your abdomen begins to swell on one side rather than evenly. This is due to the embryo developing in the tube, or to the tube becoming distended with blood. A swollen abdomen can also be a sign that the tube has ruptured and that internal bleeding is taking place. In this case there will usually be severe pain as well. You may also experience severe pain in the abdomen, or persistent pain on either side.

If the embryo dies and is reabsorbed by the body, you may notice a dull ache in your lower abdomen, and your period may be delayed by a few days.

If the embryo does continue to develop, you may experience episodes of spotting or heavier bleeding. You may also experience intermittent or continuous pain which can range from mild to severe. Sometimes the pain is a dull ache caused by internal bleeding. If the tube ruptures you may be able to feel a lump in the abdomen and go into severe shock.

Am I At Risk?

Several factors are linked with increased chance of having an ectopic pregnancy. You may be at risk if you:

- have ever suffered salpingitis – when PID affects the fallopian tubes
- have previously had a pelvic infection following miscarriage, abortion or childbirth

- have had tubal surgery, perhaps to remove blockages caused by PID
- have previously suffered an ectopic pregnancy
- have suffered any STDS – thought to account for eight out of ten ectopic pregnancies in those under 25
- suffer endometriosis, which also causes scar tissue to form
- have been sterilized
- suffer from fibroids

If any of these apply to you, it's vital to see the doctor to get a definite diagnosis as soon as you suspect you may be pregnant. Conventional pregnancy tests don't always show up positive with ectopic pregnancies and it is vital that you know whether you have conceived or not. The doctor can use more sensitive pregnancy tests plus a vaginal ultrasound scan to show up where the baby is growing. Sometimes a laparoscopy may be carried out.

What Will Be Done?

Sadly, there is no way of allowing the baby to continue growing. The embryo has to be removed to prevent the tube from rupturing, and any damage already sustained has to be repaired. If the tube is badly damaged by the pregnancy it has to removed surgically (salpingectomy), and the ovary too may have to be removed. In severe cases where a rupture has actually occurred and caused damage, hysterectomy and oophorectomy (removal of the ovaries) has to be done. In this case you will have a premature menopause.

New Hope For Sufferers

The good news is that with better techniques for diagnosing ectopic pregnancy, such drastic steps are not always necessary. Doctors can now use a suction technique to draw out the fetus, or remove the affected part of the tube using the latest techniques of micro-surgery. Three to six months after the pregnancy, further microsurgery may be performed to repair the tube. There is also research being carried out looking at leaving the pregnancy to see if it will resolve of its own accord. It has been shown that when the tube is less than 2 cm across and levels of the pregnancy hormone HCG (human chorionic gonadotrophin) are low, the fetus is reabsorbed without treatment. In this case the doctor will want to keep a very close eye on you.

Even more hope lies in a new gentle method of terminating the pregnancy using a drug called methotrexate to dissolve the fetal cells and cause them to be reabsorbed by the mother's body. The technique, which can be successfully used when the tube is less than 3 centimetres in diameter, is still at the research stage at the moment, but it is hoped that it will become more widely used. The doctor threads a thin plastic tube through the vagina, uterus and fallopian tube, under ultrasound guidance, and injects a tiny dose of the drug into the embryo. The technique is not only less traumatic than surgery, both physically and emotionally, but it also cuts the risk of scarring caused by surgery, thereby reducing the risk of subsequent infertility. However, where the tube has been damaged, surgery may again be ultimately necessary to remove scarring in some cases.

Will I Ever Have A Baby?

It has to be said that once you have suffered one ectopic pregnancy, your chances of suffering another one are raised. However, there is some good news. The most recent studies have shown that women under 30, those who were using an IUD at the time of the ectopic pregnancy, and those who were treated with conservative microsurgery (in which the tube is left in place) were more likely to have a normal subsequent pregnancy. In a study carried out in Israel it was discovered that following microsurgery 56 per cent of women with two tubes, and 46 per cent of those with one tube, went on to have a normal pregnancy. Most of these women became pregnant in the first year after the operation. And the authors of the study advise that women should try to conceive again without delay.

Infertility

PID can be responsible for both primary infertility – when you have never been able to conceive at all – and for secondary infertility, when you have had one or more children but then become infertile. Scar tissue caused by infection acts like cling film, sticking the pelvic organs together and blocking the tubes. In one report on women seeking IVF – test tube treatment – of 212 women, 176 had tubal disease and, of those, 100 had signs of previous infection with chlamydia.

Despite the dramatic advances in high-tech procedures for helping infertile couples, infertility treatment on the whole is still a bit of a hit and miss affair. Investigations can be lengthy and treatment too can be difficult, time-consuming, and hard to cope with emotionally.

The good news is that treatment for infertility caused by scarring and blocked tubes has been revolutionized in the last few years by the advent of new surgical techniques. In the past, ordinary surgery had a success rate of about 20 per cent in unblocking damaged fallopian tubes. Today, using microsurgery, success can be as high as 60 per cent, depending on the expertise of the surgeon. However, it must also be pointed out that there is a 5 to 20 per cent risk of ectopic pregnancy following tubal surgery for damage caused by PID. The success rate for microsurgery is highest in the year following surgery. It can take longer, however, as this story from the British PID Newsletter shows:

'I started my troubles in 1983. My tale is too long to recount but it was a matter of being tossed from urologist to gynaecologist before it was discovered I had massive adhesions all over the pelvic area. Anyway, we were trying for a baby and because of the adhesions my tubes were pulled out of position, so I had them cut and stitched up into position. Usually success for this op is in the first year but it took me two years, during which time I was signed on the IVF programme. However, I didn't need it – I become pregnant, and my baby is now 20 months old. The pregnancy did not make any difference to the problem, so a hysterectomy is still on the cards. I now have to decide whether to have another baby (if possible, as I was very lucky to have her) or the op.'

Recently a new technique has been developed in which a tiny balloon is inserted into the tubes and, once it is in place, blown up to keep the walls apart. The technique is still in its infancy and no one knows how successful it will prove to be, but early results seem promising.

Getting Help

If you have had PID and are experiencing trouble conceiving, it is vital to get help as soon as possible. The sooner investigations are carried out to track down the cause of problems, the sooner you can get treatment. This is important since the only option may be assisted conception techniques such as IVF – the test tube baby technique. There are often long waiting lists for such treatment, and because success rates are better in younger women, many centres refuse to take on those over a certain age (the precise age varies from centre to centre but can be as early as over 35).

The first step is to visit your GP. If you have a history of pelvic inflammatory disease, or have suffered any sexually transmitted diseases, it is worth pointing this out, as the doctor may want to refer you straight away to a specialist. Once investigations have been done to see why you are having trouble conceiving, treatment can begin.

Infertility investigations and treatment can be very wearing emotionally and you need as much support and back-up as you can get at this time. Some infertility clinics have counsellors; alternatively you can contact one of the self-help groups set up for infertile couples. For example: CHILD, PO Box 154, Hounslow, Middlesex TW5 0EZ; ISSUE – the National Fertility Association, Birmingham Settlement, 318 Summer Lane, Birmingham B19 3RL. These are also a useful source of information as to the best doctors and hospitals to go to for treatment.

IVF – In Vitro Fertilization

If your tubes are so badly damaged by scar tissue that you are unsuitable for surgery, you may decide to opt for IVF. The technique was originally developed to help this very problem, though now its use has been extended to cover women suffering other types of infertility.

The procedure involves stimulating ovulation using fertility drugs. The eggs are then collected by means of a laparoscopy and mixed with washed samples of sperm in a glass container. The fertilized embryos are then cultured in strictly controlled temperature conditions and transferred into the uterus when they are at the four cell stage – about 48 hours later. Sometimes more than one egg is implanted, because this increases the chance of one of them 'taking'. The chances of success depend partly on your age and on the skill and expertise of the doctor. At present the pregnancy rate is around 20 to 35 per cent after each try. However, what the experts call the 'take home baby rate' is still only around 10 per cent.

Treatment can be expensive – few IVF clinics in Britain are entirely NHS funded – and disappointing. It has to be said that IVF is not suitable for those with very badly scarred tubes or ovaries, since the organs may be buried so deeply that the eggs cannot be retrieved.

Coming To Terms With Infertility

If you have not conceived after four or five attempts at IVF you may have to accept that, sadly, you may never conceive. In this case you, and your partner, need as much support as possible to help you to come to terms with your feelings of grief. Again the self-help groups can be helpful. Alternatively, it may be worth seeking out a counsellor or psychologist with a special interest in fertility problems.

Fiona's Story

'I had a copper 7 IUD fitted when I was 19, which I had changed every two or three years. Round about the age of 21 I had a particular IUD which caused me a lot of problems – falling out and so on. At that time I began to suffer a lot of pelvic pain, but I struggled on taking painkillers until someone at work persuaded me to go and see the doctor. I visited the family planning clinic, where the doctor gave me an internal which was really painful. When I told him it hurt, he said, 'I can tell if it hurts you or not. Go away and live your life.' So I did. Three months later I was in hospital with raging PID having the IUD removed, and being told that I was probably infertile. I felt devastated. Having always imagined I would have children, I had to rethink my whole life.

'After that first laparoscopy I had repeated attacks of PID every couple of months. I was full of antibiotics, and though I've not had an attack for the last couple of years, I've been left with recurrent thrush and I keep getting throat infections.

I was supposed to see a specialist to have microsurgery to unblock the tubes, and was told to go away and lose a stone in weight, because the surgery would be easier. For some reason they thought I wanted to get pregnant, and when I returned to have the surgery done I was told to go away as there was no point in doing the surgery. [Results are better when the surgery is done just before a pregnancy attempt.] I got referred to a psychotherapist to help me come to terms with my infertility. However, I was the only woman in the therapy group apart from an old age pensioner, and no one knew what I was talking about. I decided to seek private psychotherapy, and that was enormously helpful. The therapist helped me to explore the conflicts I had about being childless in this society, and in a family in which you are not a real woman unless you have children. As a result I finished the dead-end relationship I was in and got on with my life. I met a new man, and we bought a house together and decided we would like to try for a family. He knew about my previous problem, but I had been told that microsurgery might just work. I went to hospital where they removed half of one of my tubes, and took the ovaries up to compensate. They removed adhesions and cuffed the tubes back so they wouldn't seal over again. Unfortunately I didn't get pregnant, and the relationship broke up – partly, I'm sure, as a result of the stress of undergoing infertility investigations and treatment and having to make love to order. I'm now having more psychotherapy, which is helping. At some level I haven't yet come to terms with not being able to have children, and I feel very bitter and angry about being fitted with a coil at such a young age and not being told of the risks. But I'm working on it. I'm thinking of becoming a foster parent. I haven't had another attack of PID since I had the microsurgery. I'm much healthier now. I try to watch my diet, and I've cut out alcohol, tea, coffee, milk and wheat. And I'm also having acupuncture and treatment with Chinese herbs in the hope that I might yet be able to have a baby.'

Pregnancy after PID
Staying Positive

Finally, in a chapter that has focused on the negative side of PID, a story with a happy ending from the British PID Newsletter:

'Seven years ago I began to get tremendous stomach-ache and backache and a red-brown discharge. I went to my GP who, without examining me, diagnosed an ineffective contraceptive Pill and prescribed another. Needless to say, this did nothing. Around the same time, my boyfriend (now my husband) began to get some disturbing symptoms so he went to an STD clinic and was diagnosed as having non-specific urethritis. I was asked to go as a contact and was also diagnosed as having a non-specific infection which was treated with antibiotics. (I was not tested for chlamydia.) Things settled down for a while but my symptoms kept recurring, never with the acuteness which they had before but severely enough to mar the first 18 months of my marriage. Intercourse was always uncomfortable and occasionally unbearably painful. I was frequently run down, unwell and depressed. Then I changed my GP. On my first visit she was very concerned by my symptoms and referred me quickly to a gynaecologist. Within seven weeks I had a laparoscopy which diagnosed PID. I was allowed out of hospital the next day. However, the surgery seemed to reactivate my condition and I was re-admitted within 48 hours with acute PID. At least now I knew I was not neurotic; I had a genuine disease. I was informed at this time that I had severe scarring on my tubes and ovaries and might not be able to conceive.

'Life continued much the same for the next five years, with all too frequent flare-ups of PID, but slowly I learned to manage the attacks: to react promptly to the symptoms with antibiotics, rest, sleep, painkillers and a good diet.

'Then I discovered I was pregnant. This came as a tremendous surprise. We had been trying but had given up hope. My pregnancy was complicated, ending in a caesarean section after 23 hours of labour but I had a lovely, healthy and whole son. I began to feel unwell and depressed about four days later. I took this to be the baby blues and took no notice. However, ten days later at home I was getting daily visits from both doctor and midwife. I again had acute PID which was complicating my recovery from surgery. I was told that when I had the caesarean, they had spent much of the surgery trying to correct the adhesions on my tubes, ovaries and womb caused by PID. However, now this new bout of PID has ruined that and it's very doubtful that I will conceive again (but they were wrong the first time, so here's hoping).

'I now have a 20-month-old son. My attacks have definitely lessened, having only two since I had my baby. I know I am very lucky. I know many women with PID will never have a child but there is always hope.'

It's vital to look after yourself during pregnancy anyway, but it's particularly important if you are a PID sufferer. Make sure you go for regular antenatal check-ups, so any problems can be picked up at an early stage. Get plenty of rest and relaxation, and if pelvic pain is a problem, consider giving up work earlier than usual so you can get enough rest. Discuss the options for delivery at an early stage with your midwife or doctor. It may help to work out your own wishes for birth by compiling a birth plan, but be prepared to be flexible should things not turn out as you hope. Pelvic pain can be eased by using TENS (see page 105). Other things which women have found helpful include massage, aromatherapy, and acupuncture.

Chapter 8

Living With PID

The good news is that most PID sufferers do recover eventually. However, an unfortunate few suffer recurrent or chronic attacks, or long-term problems brought on by damage sustained during earlier episodes. This doesn't mean you should just lie down and die! Many women have learnt to recognize the factors which trigger off problems. And the good news is that there are plenty of things you can do to help yourself and to ensure that PID doesn't come to dominate your life.

Practicalities

Work

PID can play havoc with your working life. You may work at less than full capacity if you are plagued by constant pain. You may also be constantly having to have time off – not something to endear you to most employers. Your boss is more likely to view you sympathetically if you keep him or her informed. It can be hard to let someone know you suffer from a chronic or recurrent illness when you want to appear professional. But most people are sympathetic once they are told about the problem. And you are less likely to attract labels of malingering if the powers that be know you have a real problem, than if you keep having time off work and making constant excuses.

If you are having a lot of time off, or if your condition is really affecting your work, it may be worth considering whether you could possibly go part-time, or do more work from home. In the last resort you may have to give up your job (if you can afford to). Sometimes changing to a different, less demanding kind of work may help. And it may be worth seeking careers advice to see if you can be helped to find a type of work that would be more suitable.

Children

Looking after children is hard work at the best of times. But if you are suffering recurrent illness or constant pain it can be totally exhausting. It's important as a PID sufferer not to get overtired because this can make you more prone to an attack and can also make symptoms worse, and more difficult to recover from, during one. Enlist as much help as you can with the children. If you can afford it, consider having a mother's help, nanny or childminder to help with your children. If you can't you will have to rely on the goodwill of friends and relatives.

If you are the mother of small children, enlist your health visitor in helping you find ways of coping. She is as much concerned with your health as that of your baby, and she is there to help you.

Don't be ashamed or afraid to ask for help: most people are perfectly willing to offer it, if they know there is a real problem. And if you are able to reciprocate sometimes when you are feeling better, no one is going to feel put upon. Once your children are old enough, playgroup, nursery and school will help take them off your hands for a few hours a day. You should use this time to rest and take care of yourself rather than rushing round doing the housework, or carrying bags of heavy shopping.

A Friend In Need

Many PID sufferers speak of their overwhelming gratitude to those who have helped them struggle through bad patches. Without being a moaner, it can help to let people know how the disease affects you, and the sort of help that would be most welcome at these times.

But with the best will in the world, not all friends are good at supporting you the whole time. After all, people have troubles of their own, and however much they want to help, may not always be able to do so. This is where a support network comes in handy. Sufferers from any sort of chronic illness can feel extremely isolated. It helps to have someone you can talk to who understands how you feel without you having to explain.

Sex

PID can have a devastating effect on your sex life. If every time you make love you are in agony, it's hardly surprising if, after a while, you begin to go off the idea altogether. Experts call pain during sex dyspareunia. Fortunately you don't have to give up sex altogether – except, of course, during an active attack of PID. And the good news is that orgasm can actually be good for PID because it increases blood flow to the pelvic area, which helps healing. Experiment with different ways of making love to each other. Sex doesn't always have to involve penetration. Experiment with other ways of pleasing each other such as sensuous massage, oral sex (not if you or your partner has an active infection) and so on. Use your imagination. When you do want to make love with penetration, experiment with different positions. Those where the man enters less deeply, for example lying side by side and some of the positions in which the man enters from behind, are usually more comfortable than ones in which deep thrusting takes place.

If the problem is really affecting your relationship it may help to discuss it with your family doctor, or a counsellor (see page 61).

Diet

A good diet can have an important part to play in helping you stay well and keep healthy. Experts recommend a high protein, vitamin-rich diet as the best one for recovery. Protein, of course, is not just found in the foods – such as meat and fish – that are traditionally thought of as 'protein foods': peas, beans, nuts and seeds are all good sources too. To get the most out of your diet, eat as much fresh food as possible. And try to include at least five portions of fruit and/or vegetables in your daily diet. Eat fruit and vegetables as soon as possible after buying to maximize their vitamin content, but if you have to store them do so in a cool, dark place, where air can circulate. Vitamins B, C, E and beta-carotene (which is converted in the body into vitamin A), and the mineral zinc, are thought to be especially important in keeping the immune system in shape. You can see the foods which are rich in these in the box opposite.

In addition, some PID sufferers like to take these in supplement form, or to include a multi-vitamin and mineral supplement in their daily diet. Choose any supplement you decide to use extremely carefully, since taking large doses of isolated vitamins can cause problems. Unless you know what you are doing it is best to go for a prepared supplement, or to consult a nutritional practitioner before dosing yourself with extra vitamins.

Cutting out dairy products also seems to help some

sufferers, since milk products are mucus-producing, and the production of mucus due to inflammation is one of the problems of PID.

Fighting Foods

The following foods contain the vitamins thought to boost the immune system and promote healing:

B vitamins (including thiamin, riboflavin, niacin and vitamins B6 and B12): brown rice, whole grain cereals and bread, peas, seeds, nuts, molasses, kidneys, liver and other organ meats, spinach, leafy green vegetables, eggs, brewer's yeast, wheatgerm, avocados, raisins, herrings, mackerel, cottage cheese.

Beta carotene (converted in the body into vitamin A): red, orange, yellow and dark green fruits and vegetables including carrots, sweet potato, tomatoes, apricots, peppers, spinach and so on.

Vitamin C: fruit, especially citrus fruits and blackcurrants, and green leafy vegetables such as watercress, lettuce and so on.

Vitamin E: eggs, cereals, fruit, nuts, vegetable oils, such as olive oil, seeds and seed oils, wheatgerm.

Zinc: beef, liver, seafood, nuts, cheese, carrots, ginger, mushrooms, sunflower seeds.

Rest and Relaxation

Women often find it particularly hard to relax. If you suffer PID, however, it is especially important to make time for adequate rest and relaxation – and you shouldn't feel ashamed at taking time for yourself. Stress can precipitate an attack, and can make it harder to deal with an existing one. This needn't be the completely passive sort of relaxation where you flop down on the sofa – though if you feel like doing so, then do it. It can include more active sorts such as taking up a new hobby, learning a language, joining an evening class, taking up yoga, swimming, walking and so on. Find something you like doing, and then make time for it. You need something else in your life besides PID and you will feel better for it.

Preventing PID – A 10-Point Prevention Plan

If you have ever had PID you are more at risk of developing a subsequent attack. If you are at risk, the following 10-point prevention plan will help you avoid future attacks. Even if you are not, the rules below will help you stay healthy. Many of the rules for preventing PID are a matter of common sense. Others are the same or similar as those which apply to preventing STDs. All sexually active women should be aware of these basic health guidelines, and of the signs of PID. If you are the mother of teenage daughters, you should make sure that they know how to look after their own sexual health also. And if you have sons, they too should be aware of the part they can play in spreading PID, and know how they can avoid it.

1. Don't ignore abdominal pain. Even mild pain can be a symptom of PID.

2. Think carefully about the type of contraception you use. If you are not in a permanent relationship and think you may be at risk of PID, or if you or your partner have other partners, your best bet is a barrier method such as the cap or a condom combined with a spermicide such as nonoxynol 9, which is effective against many infections, and provides a greater degree of protection against pregnancy.

3. Take care not to introduce an infection into your vagina after any event in which your cervix has been open. After birth, miscarriage or any gynaecological procedure, avoid baths – showers are better, don't douche, avoid lovemaking with penetration, and don't use tampons until you have been given the all-clear.

   Be on the lookout for any signs of infection after an abortion, miscarriage, childbirth, or any gynaecological procedure, and visit the doctor immediately if you do develop any.

   Signs to look out for include a discharge that has an unusual colour or smell, or is more profuse than usual, or different in any way from the normal changes that take place during the menstrual cycle. Other signs are a raised temperature, cystitis-like symptoms, a general feeling of unwellness or any of the symptoms listed in Chapter 2.

4. If you do have to have treatment for any sort of infection, always make sure your partner receives treatment too.

5. If you are sexually active, you should also be on the lookout for any strange discharges, lumps, bumps, irritation or smell. Go for regular check-ups at the GU clinic, especially if you take on a new partner, or if you or your partner have sex with more than one person.

6. Pay attention to personal hygiene. Wash your genital area regularly. Don't share towels, flannels and so on.

7. Other vaginal infections can bump up the chances of PID developing, as the bacteria responsible hop on the back of the existing bacteria. Such infections are more likely when the normal bacteriological balance of the vagina is changed for any reason. This can happen during a period, if you have to take antibiotics or are on the Pill. Some women find it helps to include a cupful of vinegar in the bath occasionally. Avoid bubble baths and intimate deodorants, and wash the genitals with plain water. Go

for cotton underwear rather than nylon, and avoid nylon tights and tight nylon knickers since they tend to provide the right warm, damp conditions in which bacteria flourish. Avoid tight trousers and leggings for the same reason. Change your underwear daily.

8. When you go to the toilet, always wipe your bottom from front to back to avoid bacteria from the bowel contaminating your vagina. If you have anal sex it is particularly important to make sure your partner washes his genitals before and afterwards, or preferably uses a condom, and he should always change it before entering your vagina – never go straight from anal to vaginal sex without doing so.

9. Make sure you and your sexual partners are clean. You might consider taking a shower together, as the Japanese do, before making love – or at the least wash your hands, and get your partner to wash his penis.

10. Take care during your period – women with PID often notice symptoms first during or after a period. Avoid having unprotected sex during a period – using a condom will help prevent bacteria being forced into the upper genital tract. This also makes sound sense because of the risk of AIDS being passed on during a period. Lovemaking should be particularly gentle at this time to avoid bacteria being thrust into the uterus. Look after your health generally, eat a healthy diet, get enough rest and sleep, and avoid undue stress. If you are run down you are more vulnerable to infection.

Recurrent PID

There are two steps to managing recurrent PID. The first involves trying to work out what triggers an attack. Many women find it helps to keep a diary noting when they attacks occur and what appears to trigger them. Some women find they are prone to an attack if they miss out on sleep, or if they are overdoing things at work. Others develop one when they go on holiday. The second step involves knowing how to handle attacks and making sure they are properly treated.

Step One

Use the following checklist to help sort out what sparks off your attacks.

- Have you been working harder than usual?
- Have there been any major changes in your work or personal life lately?
- Are you worried about anything?
- Have your eating or drinking habits changed recently? For example, have you been drinking more alcohol, perhaps because it is Christmas, through stress, or because your job causes you to have to socialize a lot?
- Have you been rushing or skipping meals?
- Have your sleep patterns been disrupted for any reason, for example, travel, the birth of a new baby, stress and so on?
- Have your personal hygiene habits changed for any reason – for example, have you been away from home where it has been difficult to have regular showers?
- Have you recently taken a new sex partner?
- Could your partner have taken a new sex partner?

Step Two

- Make sure you complete any courses of antibiotics that are prescribed during an attack. If the attack is only half-treated it may become more resistant to future treatment.

- Make sure the doctor tests to find out what is causing the attack so that the right combination of antibiotics can be chosen.

- Ask the doctor what drugs are being prescribed, and if s/he offers you something which didn't work previously, let him know.

- Make sure your partner is treated – even if he has no symptoms.

- Take all symptoms seriously, however minor, and seek treatment as soon as possible.

- Rest in bed until you are feeling better.

- Abstain from sex until you are clear. During a severe attack you probably won't feel up to it anyway, but even in a mild attack it is important to be careful.

- Make sure you attend for a check-up to see that you are fully recovered.

- Avoid taking repeated courses of antibiotics, which can actually perpetuate the problem by laying your immune system so low that a new infection takes hold the minute you stop taking them.

- If you aren't satisfied that you are being treated adequately, shop around for another doctor, who will investigate why you are suffering repeated attacks. One of the PID support organizations may be able to help you.

Dealing With Persistent Pain

As I said in a previous chapter, not all doctors recognize PID as a true chronic condition. However, long-term pain is widely accepted as a result of PID. In fact it's estimated that around 15 per cent of women with PID develop chronic pain.

Doctors who don't believe the pain is a symptom of continued infection say that this pain is a result of damage already inflicted by PID. The fact remains that chronic pain is an extremely distressing symptom, but there are strategies you can learn to use to help you cope.

The first step is to have investigations to find out whether PID is the true cause of pain. Many women with pelvic pain are initially diagnosed as suffering PID, whether or not this is really the case (see Chapter 5). The second step is deciding whether to seek further treatment, or whether to try and find ways of dealing with the pain that work for you. Some things that women have found helpful include the following.

Physiotherapy and Massage

Physiotherapists have a portfolio of techniques they can call upon for the relief of pain. They include massage, TENS (see below), ultrasound and various types of heat treatment.

TENS

TENS – transcutaneous electronic nerve stimulation – involves blocking pain messages by stimulating the nerve cells with a mild electric current. Physiotherapists can apply the treatment, or you can often hire or buy a machine to use at home. It consists of a box with two leads attached to two small pads which you attach to the area serving the pelvic nerves. This can be on the abdomen or the back. You are able to regulate the current by pressing the button on a small hand-held unit. The current is felt as a gentle tingling or prickling sensation, which serves to block the pain.

Ultrasound

Some physiotherapists and pain clinics have found ultrasound treatment helpful in relieving pelvic pain. The transducer – the 'arm' of the ultrasound machine which transmits sound vibrations – is held over the pelvic region and the sound vibrations act at cellular level to break up scar tissue quite painlessly.

Heat

Warmth often improves all sorts of pain. It encourages blood flow, which helps healing, and also feels soothing. Some PID sufferers swear by a holiday in a warm country to help clear up an attack. Try placing a hot water bottle, covered to prevent burning, against your abdomen, or you can buy special heating pads from camping shops and some chemists.

Sitz baths, in which you sit up to your waist in water, are soothing. Use an ordinary bath – but don't use soap or bath products in it. Alternatively, try using a baby's bath.

Another technique which helps some sufferers is called pelvic diathermy – which can be offered by a physiotherapist and some alternative practitioners such as naturopaths. A diathermy unit, which produces waves of electrical energy, is used to direct heat deep into the body's tissues. However, some women find the treatment doesn't suit them, and actually makes symptoms worse.

Acupuncture

Many women with chronic pain caused by PID have been helped by acupuncture. Widely used in China as a complete system of medicine, acupuncture is more commonly recognized in this country for its pain-relieving effects. Needles are placed in points that serve various areas of the body. It doesn't hurt but you may experience a dull, numb feeling or tingling sensation. Symptoms may disappear gradually, or get temporarily worse before getting better. You may feel tired after treatment.

It's not known exactly how acupuncture works to alleviate pain. One theory is that it blocks pain messages from reaching the brain by stimulating large nerve fibres. Others say that acupuncture stimulates the release of endorphins – the body's natural pain-relieving substances. Some recent research says that acupuncture has an anti-inflammatory effect, which could make it especially useful in treating PID.

Some doctors offer acupuncture, and many pain clinics offer it as part of their portfolio of treatments. Alternatively, you can seek private treatment from a qualified lay therapist. (For further information see Chapter 9, Alternative Ways with PID.)

Relaxation and Visualization

Relaxation is widely recognized as a way of dealing with any sort of pain. Although you can teach yourself from a book or a tape, it is probably worth seeking someone who can help teach you. There are various techniques. In some you concentrate on each muscle group in turn and relax by tightening each set of muscles and then relaxing them. In others some catchphrase is used to trigger the relaxation response. For example, you might repeat phrases to yourself such as 'My hand is getting heavy. My arm is getting heavy' and so on, again working your way through each muscle group until your whole body is relaxed. Other techniques, derived from yoga and meditation, require you to concentrate on a particular word or object while at the same time gradually becoming aware of your breathing. Slow deep breathing can sometimes help you relax.

Visualization is a technique culled from meditation and yoga in which you imagine your body getting better. The technique has been widely used in the treatment of cancer and chronic pain of all kinds. The idea is to get into a state of deep relaxation and then to imagine your body healing itself or the pain ebbing away. You might visualize your pain as a hard piece of ice and then see it melting in the warm sun. Alternatively you might see it as a centre of darkness and imagine it becoming flooded with healing light. Pick an image and use what feels right to you.

However, do be aware that simply thinking positive can't help in all cases, and don't feel guilty or a failure if it doesn't work for you.

Chapter 9

Alternative Ways
With PID

Many women find it helpful to combine orthodox medical
and self-help approaches to PID with alternative, or as many
practitioners prefer to call it, complementary medicine.

Seeking out alternative healthcare can make you feel as
though you are more in control of your illness, whereas when
you are being processed through the orthodox medical system
it is easy to feel completely powerless. As you find your way
through the various alternative treatments, and try to choose
the one that is best for you, you can feel a renewed sense of
purpose, which in itself can be emotionally and mentally
healing, as the following account shows.

Margaret's Story

'I got so tired with all the toing and froing to the doctor and
the antibiotics I was constantly on that I decided to try
alternative therapies. At first I visited a homoeopath. I was
prescribed lachesis for the sharp pain, caulophyllum for
cervical contractions and belladonna for the period pain. The
homoeopath was wonderful – for the first time there was
someone who took me seriously. She was always there on the
end of a phone. She got me to grade my pain on a scale of

0-10 and to tell her what it was. If it got over 5 I was to ring the doctor.

'After seeing the homoeopath I started going every week for a massage, and that was really helpful in soothing the pain and reducing my level of stress. After a while she also did Shiatsu massage, and used a moxa stick, in which a roll of the herb St John's Wort is burned and applied to the acupuncture points.

'Two years ago I started to undergo Gestalt Therapy. I was taught how to do visualization, which I did for 20 minutes, three times a day. The therapist explained that it didn't mean pretending that everything was well. She asked me to describe to her exactly what I thought was happening in my body. I described the adhesions, and said that during ovulation green slime comes from my womb. She then asked me to imagine a team of tiny people going round cleaning my womb. I fantasized all these tiny people with little brooms and space helmets on their heads. Next I fantasized the team in the left fallopian tube with feather brushes dipping them in olive oil and cleaning and soothing the fallopian tube on the left-hand side. After six weeks I stopped bleeding. Previous to that I had been losing black blood from my period to ovulation, and then fresh red blood from ovulation to my period, and then my period would be enormously heavy. It sounds incredible but when I had the laparoscopy there were no adhesions on the left-hand side at all.

'Next I changed to a holistic GP who encourages you to read your notes and negotiate on equal terms. This doctor accepted immediately that I was ill and at a stroke removed a big barrier to me getting well by issuing me with a three month sick note. It was huge relief to be believed and to be given permission to be ill.

'He also discovered that I had candida as well as PID. I was very fat – I looked about 8 months pregnant. He put me on a strict anti-candida diet, and I felt tons better and began to take an interest in what I could do with my life.

'After a while, as the physical symptoms began to improve, I began to go to pieces mentally. I had terrible nightmares and daydreams and that was when I went into therapy. It was then that I discovered that I had been sexually abused as a child, but I had squashed down all the memories. As I opened up each new incident a symptom seemed to disappear. Today I'm almost symptom-free.'

Finding the therapy or combination of therapies that suits you is largely a matter of trial and error. It can help to talk to other women who have tried alternative treatments to see what helped them. But bear in mind that because most alternative treatments look at the individual rather than the illness, what suited one person may not be right for you.

How Can Alternative Therapies Help?

Most alternative therapies work on the underlying principle of boosting the body's own recuperative powers. They aim to support the body in such a way that its own healing mechanisms can begin to swing into action. Such an approach is attractive because it seems gentler than the traditional medical approach with its emphasis on powerful drugs and surgery. That's not to say that these approaches don't have an extremely valuable part to play in treating PID. Acute PID is a serious illness – and serious illnesses are what orthodox medicine does best. However, recurrent and chronic sufferers may prefer to look beyond the conventional medical approach to see what alternative therapies can have to offer.

Alternative healthcare attempts to look at you as a whole person. The practitioner will take time to find out about you, your lifestyle and relationships. Many orthodox practitioners don't take these things into account, and yet if you have a chronic condition, learning how to deal with it within the context of your individual lifestyle is one of the most important things. Most alternative therapists are able to spend longer with you than the average ten minutes of so of the typical GP consultation.

Many women complain of the brusqueness and impersonality of orthodox medical consultants. They feel that as far as the doctor is concerned, they are little more than a set of reproductive organs with a pair of legs attached. And though this attitude may be unfair to some doctors, it's a sad fact that most medical practitioners don't have to time to get to know their patients and relate to them as people. Another plus point for some women is that while most doctors are men, most alternative practitioners are women, with the exception of a couple of alternative therapies such as osteopathy and chiropractic. There are more alternative practitioners and more choice of therapies, so if you feel you would prefer a woman therapist it may be easier to shop around until you have found one.

Which Therapy?

Almost any of the alternative therapies can help PID sufferers, but the following may be particularly useful.

Homoeopathy

Homoeopathy involves treating patients with minute doses of substances that in a well person would produce the symptoms of the illness being treated. Although no one knows exactly why this should work, many people swear by it. Certainly, homoeopathy is one of the gentlest forms of therapy. The active substances in the remedies are in such minute quantities that they can't possibly do any harm.

Choosing A Homoeopath

There are two sorts of homoeopath: those who are medically trained, and lay homoeopaths who have undergone extensive training in homeopathy. Because PID is a complex illness, you may feel happier seeing a practitioner who is also medically qualified, but it may be more difficult to find one. If you do decide to seek treatment from a lay homoeopath, make sure you see one who is properly trained (see useful addresses at the end of this chapter). You should preferably choose a practitioner who has a special interest in PID or in treating women's ailments. Ask the practitioner if he or she has treated anyone with your condition before. It may even be possible for the practitioner to put you in touch with such a patient, who can tell you how effective the treatment was for her. Alternatively, the PID Support Network may be able to help you find a suitable practitioner.

What Will Happen When You Visit A Homoeopath?

Homoeopaths, like all alternative practitioners, aim to treat their patients as individuals. The homoeopath will ask you a lot of questions about your illness, and also a number of what may seem strange questions about your lifestyle, tastes in food, drink, and so on. On the basis of this he or she builds up a symptom picture which is then matched to a particular remedy. Homoeopaths have a whole repertoire of remedies that they can call on, and the skill of the homoeopath lies in the ability to match the patient to the remedy as precisely as possible. For this reason it is impossible to say what particular remedy or remedies would be used to treat PID, since they will vary from person to person, depending on the picture the homoeopath builds up of them and their symptoms.

Those attending for homoeopathic treatment sometimes

experience an aggravation of their symptoms at first. However, this is usually welcomed by the homoeopath as a sign that the body is beginning to fight off the illness.

Herbal Treatment

Herbs have been used for centuries to treat and cure a whole variety of illnesses. In fact, many modern drugs are derived originally from herbal treatments.

Again, as PID is a complex illness, it is better to consult a qualified herbal practitioner – in the UK, look for the letters MNIMH (Member of the National Institute of Medical Herbalists) when choosing a practitioner to be sure the person you go to has had a proper training. It's also worth seeking out a therapist who has a particular expertise in treating women's illnesses.

What Will Happen When I Consult A Herbalist?

Consultation is much like consultation with an ordinary medical practitioner. The precise herb or combination of herbs required to treat you will vary depending on your symptoms and how widespread the problem is. But herbal practitioners can call on a wide variety of medicines for PID. These might have to be taken internally as pills or tinctures or in the form of a herbal tea, or externally as douches, compresses or packs. Treatment might include herbs to reduce inflammation, painkilling herbs, herbs which act on the female reproductive organs, such as agnus vitex castor, and herbs which help boost the immune system, such as echinacea.

The herbalist will advise you on diet and other lifestyle measures that can help banish infection.

It is especially important to keep your doctor informed if

you are taking any herbal remedies, and to inform your herbal practitioner of any orthodox remedies you are taking, since herbs can react with or against some of the constituents found in drugs.

Aromatherapy

Aromatherapy, which uses essential oils derived from aromatic plants, flowers, seeds and barks, is a particularly attractive therapy to many women. Most aromatherapists are themselves women.

Many oils have powerful anti-infective properties, while others seem to act more at a mental level to soothe or arouse. The actual treatment consists of using the oils in massage or in baths. The oils are absorbed into the circulation where they act via the nervous or hormonal system. Research is at present going on in some British NHS hospitals to see whether it is the scents of the oils, or the massage component of aromatherapy which has the most beneficial effect.

Aromatherapy may be particularly useful for PID because some oils are extremely good at healing scarring. Massage is a very effective treatment for many kinds of pain. Oils that might be used include tea tree, which is known to be especially successful against infections of the genital tract and as an immune system booster, lavender, a good all-purpose oil, and rosewood or palmarosa oils.

Acupuncture, Acupressure And Shiatsu

Acupuncture has already been mentioned for its helpfulness in relieving the pain of PID. But it can also be used to help tone and rebalance the system. Recent research has shown acupuncture to help boost the body's resistance to inflammation and to boost the production of white blood cells, the body's first line of defence against infection.

Acupressure and shiatsu are different types of

acupuncture, without the needles. Pressure is exerted by the fingers, or other parts of the therapist's body, on the appropriate acupuncture points. The therapies are particularly good at relieving pain and treating stress. And they can be learnt to use yourself at home for quick pain relief without drugs.

Nutritional Therapies and Naturopathic Medicine

We've seen how a healthy diet can help you resist infection and stay healthy. We've also seen that the body is more prey to infection with PID if the immune system is below par. The nutritional therapies take this one step further by using dietary means to treat and prevent illness.

Recurrent infections are seen by nutritional practitioners as a sign that the body's natural balancing mechanisms are out of sync. Repeated courses of antibiotics and the Pill are seen as contributing to this lack of balance.

Naturopaths make use of a variety of detoxification techniques such as fasting, enemas, raw foods and juices and so on to help clear the body of poisons which are thought to cause disease, so that the immune system can begin to function properly again. Naturopathic practitioners may also recommend hydrotherapy – treatment with water. We all know how soothing sitting in a warm bath can be for aches and pains. Naturopaths take this one stage further by using hot and cold water to stimulate the circulation to the affected area in order to promote healing. You may be advised to sit in a sitz bath (hip bath) of cold water, while keeping the rest of the body warmly clothed.

Other nutritional therapists use vitamin supplements to boost the system and help fight illness.

For pelvic inflammatory disease a wholefood diet, with plenty of raw leafy and root vegetables, nuts, seeds, and a little fresh milk and fish roe may be recommended.

Jane's Story

'After years of unsatisfactory treatment with conventional medicine and antibiotics, I decided to try alternative therapies. First of all I visited a naturopath who put me on a detoxifying diet of fresh fruit and vegetables. I also had to avoid meat, alcohol, coffee and curries. After that I visited a practitioner in Chinese Medicine who treated me with acupuncture and Chinese herbs. He examined me and took various pulses. He then asked me several questions that seem quite strange to anyone who is used to visiting a conventional doctor, such as how the weather affected me, likes and dislikes, and whether I preferred hot to cold. In Chinese terms PID is due to a yang deficiency, and is associated with cold and dampness. At first I had to attend every three weeks for acupuncture. The treatment took about 20 minutes and the needles were inserted into my abdomen, ankles, wrist and lower back. I also had to take a variety of herbs to strengthen the body and detoxify it of the damage done by the antibiotics. I felt tremendously calmer immediately. After a year I started to feel completely well again, and today I only need to go once every six months to have acupuncture to rebalance my energy. I've only had one course of antibiotics since I started the therapy, and I feel much better for it.'

Mind-Body Therapies

There is often a large psychological component in PID. To admit this is not to suggest that the illness is 'all in the mind', or that you are 'imagining it'. Research has shown that depression, anxiety and other emotional upsets can actually depress the immune system, making you more vulnerable to illness. And we've also seen that many women find that being under stress can spark off an attack of PID or make existing symptoms worse. Psychotherapy can take various forms. It can include techniques such as visualization – a technique culled from yoga, and various other techniques to help you get in touch with your feelings and feel more relaxed.

Biofeedback
This is an extension of relaxation technique. Electrodes are used to measure signs of stress such as changes in body temperature, heart rate and so on, that can show whether or not you are relaxed. You are then taught simple relaxation techniques and are able to monitor how relaxed you are. After a while you will learn to produce the relaxation response without the need for the biofeedback machine.

Yoga
Many sufferers find yoga helpful at easing the pain. It's a particularly gentle form of exercise, and also works at the mind level.

Useful Addresses

To find an alternative or complementary practitioner:
The Institute for Complementary Medicine
21 Portland Place
London W1
Tel 071 636 9543

Acupuncture
British Acupuncture Register and Directory
34 Alderney Street
London SW1V 4EC
Tel 071 834 1012

Council for Acupuncture
Suite 1
19a Cavendish Square
London W1M 9AD
Tel 071 495 8153

Aromatherapy
International Federation of Aromatherapists
4 East Mearn Road
London SE21 8AA
(Enclose SAE)

Tisserand Aromatherapy Institute
10 Victoria Grove
Second Avenue
Hove
E Sussex BN3 3WJ
Tel 0273 206640

Nutritional Counselling
The Dietary Therapy Society
33 Priory Gardens
London N6 5QU
Tel 081 341 7260

The Women's Nutritional Advisory Service
PO Box 268
Hove
E Sussex BN3 1RW
Tel 0273 771366

Institute for Optimum Nutrition,
5 Jerdan Place,
London SW6 1BE
Tel 071 385 7984

British Nutritional Medicine Society (as for Women's Nutritional Advisory Service).

Homeopathy
(Medical homoeopaths)
British Homoeopathic Association
27a Devonshire Street
London W1N 1JR
Tel 071 935 2163

(Lay homoeopaths)
Society of Homoeopaths
2 Artizan Road
Northampton NN1 4HU
Tel 0604 21400
or
The Hahnemann Society
Avenue Lodge
Bounds Green Road
London N22 4EU
Tel 081 889 1595

Herbalism
National Institute of Medical Herbalists
41 Hatherley Road
Winchester
Hants SO22 6RR
Tel 0962 68776

Chapter 10

Towards The Future

The good news is that after years in the shadows, doctors are becoming more aware of PID. In 1990 an editorial in the prestigious *British Medical Journal* was devoted to PID and its treatment, showing that medical consciousness of the problems is being raised.

Better Diagnosis

As the importance of chlamydia is beginning to be recognized, scientists are working on devising simpler, more sensitive and accurate tests for detecting the infection. Diagnosis of PID should become better too as doctors become more aware of the usefulness of laparoscopy. In the UK, changes in the GPs' contract encouraging them to conduct regular check-ups, and better diagnostic facilities in their surgeries, should lead to GPs becoming more experienced in treating sexually transmitted infections and make it easier to get diagnosis and treatment at an early stage. New methods of diagnosis such as vaginal ultrasound mean that detection of PID, and problems caused by it such as ectopic pregnancy, will become easier too.

Better Treatment

The increased awareness of PID and chlamydia is leading to more research into the best methods of treating them. New antibiotics are being tried out, and experiments into the best regimens for treating the various forms of PID are being worked out. Hope lies too in better treatment for some of the serious long-term consequences of PID.

Work is going on to improve IVF techniques; new methods of terminating ectopic pregnancies mean that losing the tube is not an inevitable consequence. Research is also going on into ways of alleviating long-term pain caused by adhesions.

More Understanding

The best news of all is that many doctors are beginning to understand that women complaining of pelvic pain are not simply malingerers or neurotic. The discovery that pelvic congestion is a reality has led doctors to take women complaining of pelvic pain more seriously, and this should have a knock-on effect in the diagnosis of PID, since doctors are more likely to send women for further investigations to get to the root of the pain.

Better Information

One good outcome of AIDS/HIV is that we are all becoming much more aware of the importance of safe sex. More people are turning to barrier methods of contraception which, as we have seen, can protect against PID, as well as HIV and cervical cancer.

Thinking Positive

Finally PID, like any serious or chronic illness, can actually bring about positive changes in your life. Coming to terms with a long-term illness, or with infertility, can change your way of experiencing things, and cause you to look at life in a new, more positive way. Even a simple step like joining a self-help group and discovering that you are not alone can be enormously helpful. In the end, each woman has to find her own way out of the shadows, but it can be done.

Margaret, the language teacher who was dogged for seven years with recurrent attacks of acute PID (see Chapter 2 and Chapter 9), has now retired on health grounds and is training to be a psychotherapist. She says, 'I took up art and I started to put myself first for a change. This month I have two paintings in an exhibition. I look after myself. I eat properly, I go for massage, I make sure I get enough rest and exercise. In short, I care for myself in a way I didn't before. My life is full and rich.'

Libby, who suffered nine years of constant pain and agony, and was declared sub-fertile (see chapter 5), now has a baby, and says, 'I have come to terms with my PID. At one time my life was ruled by PID – today I feel I am in control of it. I've stopped looking for cures and learnt to manage it. I know my limitations and what I can and can't do. I try to be sensible and get help with shopping and housework. I take painkillers if the pain is really severe, but other than that I have found that a hot water bottle and rest helps. I'm getting on with my life. I'm doing a sociology course at night school, and that's an interest. I'm much more positive.'

Jane, who finally threw out all her antibiotics and started being treated with acupuncture (see Chapters 6 and 9) says, 'I feel tremendously calmer now. It took a year before I started to feel better, but today I'm virtually free of attacks. I've got a part-time job and life feels good.'

Paula, who has been plagued with pelvic pain since she was in her teens says, 'You feel terribly isolated, as if you are the only one. But since joining the PID Support Network I've become much more positive. At one time I used to think I've got a pain, and it would be the end of the world. I would spend days indoors or come home from work early. Now I take the attitude that what I've got isn't going to kill me. It's something I've got to live with. I've found ways of dealing with the pain. I find raspberry leaf tea helps to relax me, or a hot water bottle. In the last couple of years I've tried to push it out of my mind.'

PID Support Network

This is an association of sufferers, founded by former sufferer Jessica Pickard, which exists to inform and support women with PID. The Network has no formal structure, and there are no groups as such, as women with PID are often unable to get out of the house for meetings because of their condition. Instead, women in various areas act as supporters to fellow sufferers. The Network produces an excellent newsletter, which details latest research and information, and includes personal stories from sufferers.

PID Support Network
c/o Women's Health Research and Information Centre
52-54 Featherstone Street
London EC1Y 8RT
Tel 071-251 6580/6332

Index

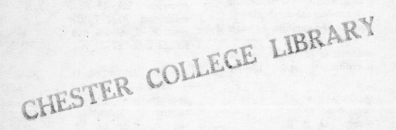